steps to fight

Chronic Fatigue Syndrome

For The Modern Woman

Dr. A.W. Martin D.C., Ph.D.

Contents

Introduction

For the past 15 years I have watched in horror as a new syndrome has developed from nothing to a national disaster. When I was in school, diseases such as AIDS and Chronic Fatigue Syndrome did not exist. Now, one out of every four visits to the doctor in North America are from people suffering from Chronic Fatigue Syndrome or Fibromyalgia. This book is a culmination of 15 years of personal research on Chronic Fatigue Syndrome. I have monitored over 500 people for the last several years suffering from this terrible epidemic.

The Center for Disease Control in Atlanta, Georgia tells us that 90 million people worldwide suffer from Chronic Fatigue Syndrome. <u>Well over 80% of these people are women</u>. This book is written with a great amount of passion. Why? - because my wife and literally hundreds of my patients have fallen victim to this new syndrome. Friend, when a disorder like this hits close to home you want to help others understand that this disease is not in your head, although, as you will read later, many of the areas in the brain are affected. I also want you to know that there is help out there!

I hope you will find this book informative and a real blessing. I have tried not to make it too complicated. I used the KISS method: **KEEP IT SIMPLE STUPID!** As you read this book I hope that you will appreciate that Chronic Fatigue Syndrome is a multi-symptom syndrome. Several chapters will show the connection that stress, depression, parasites, hypoglycemia, yeast, allergies and even cancer have with Chronic Fatigue Syndrome (CFS).

I will show you how CFS affects almost every organ in the body. You will then start to understand the domino effect this has on every system in the body, including the nervous, endocrine, hormonal and especially the body's immune system. One of the big problems with CFS is misdiagnosis. It amazes me how some doctors still fail to recognize this disorder in spite of literally hundreds of books and professional papers written on the subject. By the way, one of Dr. Death's (Jack Kevorkian-not one of my favourite people) assisted suicides was with a patient who was suffering from CFS. You can imagine how sick this poor lady felt.

I would like to dedicate this book to the late Dr. Rudy Falk, MD. Dr. Falk was a pioneer in medicine. He was a cancer specialist who admitted that modern medicine does not have all of the answers. He was open to anything that might help his patients. I would also like to express my thanks to Dr. Zoltan Rona who is one of the most brilliant men that I have ever met.

I want to thank my wife Rose-Marie who did the lion's share of the work on this manuscript. It always amazes me how well she functions in spite of having CFS. I would also like to give glory to my Lord and Saviour, Jesus Christ who came into my life in 1982.

PART 1

The Problem:

Chronic Fatigue Syndrome

The New Epidemic

C H A P T E R   O N E

CFS - The New Epidemic

"Something has happened since 1985". I have said this over and over again in several hundred radio and TV interviews. Why this answer? Well it is in response to the question - Why are people so sick and tired today? I have noticed a dramatic shift in my own practice and experience. I have a Ph.D. in nutrition and have been a practising chiropractor since 1974. I can tell you from my collected clinical statistics that since 1985 people are not getting healthier, but are actually worse than ever. Do you know in the early 1970's, one woman in 20 developed breast cancer, but today it is one out of every eight. Men have not done any better. In 1974 one out of every 15 men after the age of 50 had a chance of developing prostate cancer. Now it is one out of four. My word!! What is happening? Before 1985 one out of 20 children came into my office with asthma and allergies. Since 1985, one out of 3 kids in my clinic have asthma or allergies. [1]

Here Is A List of Diseases That Have Increased In Frequency Since 1985: [2]

• Chronic Fatigue Syndrome
• Breast Cancer
• Stomach Cancer
• Asthma and Allergies
• Diabetes and Hypoglycemia
• Attention Deficit Disorder
• Manic Depression

In this book I will set out to prove that even though we are spending millions of dollars on so called health care, **we are not getting healthier.** Oh sure, on average we are living a little longer but we are certainly not in better shape. What is happening? Why are we so tired? Why are diseases like Chronic Fatigue Syndrome and Attention Deficit Disorder out of control? Why are Asthma and Diabetes on a record increase? Is there a link between all of the diseases?

Three Reasons For Declining Health In Women

In the last 15 years there has been a major shift in women's health. The Center for Disease Control in Atlanta, Georgia tells us that there are over 90 million people world wide suffering from Chronic Fatigue Syndrome.[3]   One out of every four visits to doctors in North America are from people suffering from Chronic Fatigue. There are three categories of causes which explain why women are so worn out today. This world, especially North America has changed dramatically in the last 15 years!!

Lifestyle

In the last 15 years, a record number of women have joined the work force. The average working woman spends eight hours a day at work and then comes home and works again. Guess what ladies, your body was not made to do this. It was not until my wife, a registered nurse, registered nutritional consultant, and mother of our four children, got sick that I clued into how hard women work. Hello!!! Men are so dense. When my wife took ill in 1991 with Chronic Fatigue Syndrome, I was forced to take over some of her regular duties. How do women do it? She worked all day with me at the office and then started her second job at home. No wonder women are getting sick. No wonder they are burnt out! The average woman works twice as hard as men. I mean, I work hard, but when I go home I relax. I helped out with the children, but nothing in comparison to what my wife did. Ladies, your bodies were not meant to work 16-18 hours a day!!

Stress

Who is not stressed today? According to statistics, the number one problem that doctors see in their office today is stress.[4] People are under enormous amounts of pressure which is different today in so many ways compared to the past. I will spend time in chapter five on what stress does to our body's immune system and the effect that it has on Chronic Fatigue Syndrome. In the meantime study after study has confirmed that the immune system gets broad-sided by undue stress. For example, if someone is going through a divorce, separation or has lost a spouse, their chances of getting cancer or having a stroke is increased by 50-60% in their first year.[5]

Nutritional

What has changed in last 15 years as far as our diets are concerned? Again, we do not have to put our brains on auto-pilot to figure this one out! Fast foods have become a major part of our eating patterns. Fast foods are loaded with saturated fats and lacks the nutrients one needs to keep healthy. Another factor is that we consume far too much sugar. We would not consider putting sugar into our gas tanks, so why do we insist on putting sugar into our blood-stream. It does a lot of harm. As a matter of fact, as I will explain later, sugar is a major contributor to heart disease, cancer and a host of other diseases.

Probably the number one reason that people are not as healthy today as before is the lack of fiber in our diets. The average woman needs at least 30-40 grams of fiber daily.[6] However, most women in the western world eat between 5-10 grams a day. Why is fiber so important? Did you know that there is a direct link between the lack of fiber in a woman's diet and breast cancer. A woman who is chronically constipated has a 40-50% increase in chances of developing breast cancer!! Why? When women do not eliminate toxins from their bodies, the toxins are reabsorbed through their lymphatic system and poison the breast tissue. Do you want to know why we are losing the war on breast cancer? Why have women been dying more and more frequently in the last 15 years from this dreaded disease? **Lack of fiber in their diets; pure and simple!!** In the meantime the American Cancer Society slogan that "Cancer can be beaten" is attractive but in reality, far from the truth. We literally spend millions of dollars on research each year to find the so called genetic cause of cancer, while we are losing the war on breast cancer. Ladies, start by **preventing** breast cancer. By the way, do not get me started on the Cancer Society's so called prevention of breast cancer. Their idea of prevention is called early detection. But ladies, if you find a lump on your breast it is already too late!! Any doctor worth his salt knows that a palpable lump is already 5-10 years old. That means that the cancer has already started to damage the body. Winning the war on cancer is preventing cancer, pure and simple.

Environmental

Once again, one need not have graduated with a PhD to realise that our environment has drastically changed in the last 15 years. My heavens, Ralph Nader recently wrote that the average drinking water supply in major US cities contains over 2100 chemicals.[7] Imagine all the crap that eventually ends up in our bodies. No wonder why we are so sick!!! Can you eat a piece of meat nowadays that has not been pumped full of antibiotics and hormones? There are so many herbicides and pesticides used today on our soil which makes most soil dangerously low in essential minerals. The average apple has 25% less vitamin C than an apple from the same orchard 25 years ago.

Do you see the pattern developing now? Our lifestyle, our nutrition and our environment have contributed to the increase in a serious number of diseases. **Friend, we are not getting healthier, but worse by the minute.**

Fatigue - A Symptom or Start of Something More Serious

Everybody gets tired, but to always be tired and to never have very much energy is a sign that your body is not functioning well. Ladies, if you have a lack of energy, listen to your body, it is trying to tell you something. You may be starting a major problem such as Chronic Fatigue Syndrome.

Diagnostic Criteria For Chronic Fatigue Syndrome

In this chapter, I want to explain everything that is known about CFS. I will also explain the differences between CFS and Fibromyalgia.

If you are just starting to go through the battery of tests, but you suspect that you do have CFS or FMS, be forewarned; routine laboratory testing reveals nothing about CFS or FMS. Since fatigue and pain are individual and cannot be seen, measured or spotted in a blood test, the problem is often downplayed. <u>The blood of CFS patients' is invariably statistically no different from that of healthy control subjects and if abnormality cannot be found, doctors may think the symptoms are imaginary.</u> Just be aware that this is not the Yuppie Flu and the <u>depression </u>comes "after being sick and tired of being sick and tired".

These following criteria are from the Center of Disease Control guidelines published in the Annuals of Internal Medicine.

Symptoms of Chronic Fatigue Syndrome [8]

• Fatigue (persistent, not relieved by rest, lasts for at least six or more consecutive months)

• Tender cervical or axillary nodes in neck region

• Sleep disorder (though extremely fatigued, sleep may only last one to two hours or 10-12 hours of unrefreshed, dream-filled sleep)

• Cognitive or memory impairment (difficulty in concentrating, confusion, thick heavy fog over the brain especially during the tired times, dizzy spells)

• Chronic sore throat (may not show signs of infection)

• Muscle pain, multi-joint pain (but not arthritis)

• Allergies (Environmental and food sensitivities)

• Irritable bowel (alternating between diarrhea and constipation)

• New onset headaches (tension-type or migraine)

• Post-exertional malaise (fatigue, pain and flu-like symptoms after exercise)

One need not have all these symptoms to have CFS. In my experience, these are the 4 most prevelant symptoms of CFS:

1) Fatigue
2) Cognitive or memory impairment
3) Sleep disorder
4) Muscle pain

Comparison of Chronic Fatigue Syndrome and Fibromyalgia

CHRONIC FATIGUE SYNDROME	FIBROMYALGIA
• Fatigue - major complaint in CFS	• Fatigue - not as severe as in CFS
• Muscle Pain - generalized aches and muscle pain - not as debilitating as in fibromyalgia.	• Muscle Pain - the major complaint in fibromyalgia patients. Specific multi-joint pain and muscle aches- one muscle group constantly aches more than any other muscle group
• Memory Loss - all CFS patients experience cognitive and memory problems	• Memory Loss - not all patients experience memory problems
• Allergies skin, chemical, food and environmental allergies are common in CFS	• Allergies not as prevalent in fibromyalgic patients as in CFS

• Stress (internal) - usually starts after a lengthy history of antibiotic use or stress over an extended period of time (ie: family problems, divorce, or death of a spouse)

Stress - usually starts after severe trauma (ie: whiplash injury from a car accident)

• Sleep disorder - falling asleep and staying asleep is characteristic, alternating with 10-12 hours sleeping and waking up unrefreshed. General complaint among CFS sufferers - "I can't fall asleep because my brain won't turn off"

• Sleep disorder - Difficulty in sleeping because of fibromyalgic pain

Noteworthy:

Five of the nine criteria relate to pain and are often present in Fibromyalgia as well. According to the Center of Disease Control you will not be diagnosed as a CFS patient if you have any other co-existing medical condition. On the other hand FMS is a distinct clinical entity that stands on its own, regardless of whether a person has other medical problems. This may be why you hear of more FMS diagnosis (2% of the general population) as compared to CFS (roughly 0.5% of the general population). This disease is so prevalent that the Center for Disease has established a special hotline for CFS sufferers.[9]

Just let me start out by saying that I have never seen a patient with true Chronic Fatigue Syndrome that does not have Fibromyalgia, and a Fibromyalgia patient that does not have Chronic Fatigue Syndrome. An internist tends to diagnosis his patient with Chronic Fatigue Syndrome and a Rheumatoligist will diagnosis fibromyalgia.

Between 1984-87, the number of patients appearing in a doctor's office with CFS symptoms doubled and between 1987-89, the numbers doubled yet again.[10] Doctors who have done very little studying on the subject are sceptical and choose to believe that CFS does not really exist, declaring it to be depression and patients end up on antidepressants, painkillers, and tranquillizers. These drugs do very little to treat the disorder and may actually do a lot of harm.

New Cases Of CFS Per Year

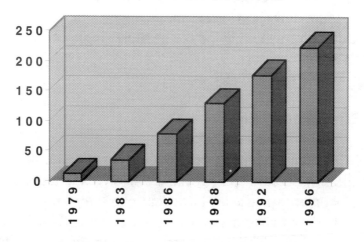

A New Disorder

I want everyone to know that Chronic Fatigue Syndrome is a new disorder. Just like Aids, this syndrome has been in existence since the late 70's and early 1980's. This is not a burn out. This is not simply people having a bad hair day. CFS, as you will see, is very serious and has it's own unique set of symptoms.

Possible Causes of CFS

1) Long Term Antibiotic Use

Time and time again we've noticed that well over 80% of people who suffer from Chronic Fatigue Syndrome have had a long history of antibiotic use. So often we notice that CFS sufferers had frequent recurrences of middle ear or throat infections during their infancy. Dr. Michel Rosebaum and Dr. Murray Susser suggest that antibiotic treatment for acne may be the greatest single contributor to CFS.[11]

2) Birth Control Pill

Another common thread of CFS patients was the use of the birth control pill. It has been my experience that most women who use the birth control pill for a prolonged period (over two years) suffer from chronic yeast infections (candida). This yeast infection might be low grade, meaning that quite often a woman doesn't even realize that she is suffering from it. However, a yeast infection will definitely lower the immune system over a period of time.

3) Exposure To Mold

The more we learn about Chronic Fatigue, the more I'm convinced that exposure to mold is a major culprit. Time and time again, survey after survey, I have seen a link between CFS and mold. A recent book entitled "Prevention of Cancer - Hope at Last" has shown some very interesting results concerning mold and its relationship to breast cancer. [12]

Remember, anyone that is around air conditioning is exposed to mold. Hot tubs, overly insulated homes all create a friendly environment for mold growth. Mold literally tears down an already compromised immune system.

4) Trauma

Another interesting factor that seems to be quite common amongst CFS sufferers is a traumatic event. What I'm saying is that often times a person might have been going through severe stress in a relationship such as divorce, separation or loss of a loved one. Even a car accident 2 years or so prior to onset of CFS is quite prevalent. These types of trauma no doubt compromise the immune system.

Why Is CFS So Misunderstood?

There Are Two Reasons Why CFS Has Been So Maligned:

• It happens mostly to women (over 80%).

• Most standard medical tests including blood results are usually within normal limits.

Can you see the picture now? Here's a woman who goes into a doctor's office and complains of bizarre symptoms including flu-like symptoms and severe fatigue. He orders a battery of tests and when the results come in they are basically normal. He then assumes that a person with CFS is depressed - you know, having trouble with their marriage, kids etc. So the dear doctor orders antidepressants and sleeping pills. Therefore, the merry-go-round continues.

Here's What To Do

First and foremost, try and find a doctor who specializes in Chronic Fatigue Syndrome or at least is quite sympathetic. Don't be afraid to diagnose yourself after the doctor has ruled out all other possibilities. Remember, you know more about your body than anyone else. **So take charge.** Get all the information you can and demand answers to your questions. I find it extremely helpful when patients write down their questions before they come to see me at my office. This way we don't get side tracked.

What happens far too often, because of nervousness and short term memory loss, is that you will forget to ask your doctor certain questions. Write them down and make sure they are answered to your satisfaction.

Nine Common Clinical Findings With Patients Suffering From CFS

1) Diminished Blood Flow To The Brain

Spect scan results (this new technology involves the use of two radioactive substances that cross the blood brain barrier) show diminished blood flow in the brain of CFS patients.[13] These 4 areas include the areas that influence thinking and learning.

Dr. Les Simpson, of New Zealand, suggests that most CFS patients have cupped shaped red blood cells. This has a tendency to decrease oxygen supply to the brain.[14]

2) Altered Brain Wave Patterns In Chronic Fatigue Syndrome

A researcher in Charlotte, North Carolina, Myra Preston, states that brain wave patterns seen in CFS patients are exactly opposite of the brain wave patterns of healthy people. When a healthy person is awake and functioning, the brain primarily produces a combination of alpha and beta waves. Chronic Fatigue sufferers produce a very low level of alpha and beta waves and appear to be stuck in theta waves. Theta waves simply means, that the brain is stuck in neutral. The result is that the patient is never fully awake and able to function intellectually at their optimum level. Neither can they fall deeply asleep. Preston studied 80 CFS patients and found that 95% of them produced this type of abnormality. [15]

The four types of brain wave patterns are:

- Alpha waves - a state of calm and relaxation
- Beta waves - in which intellectual functioning occurs
- Theta waves - the state of drowsiness before falling asleep
- Delta wave - the brain wave seen during deep sleep

3) Bright Lesions In The Brain

There is considerable evidence that CFS patients have similar bright spots in certain areas of the brain that are quite similar to those found in Multiple Sclerosis.[16]

4) Subclinical Hypoglycemia

I will spend a whole chapter explaining the relationship between CFS and hypoglycemia. Remember, that hypoglycemia itself is hard to diagnose, unless you have an extremely severe case. Get the standard tests done, but if you have CFS then you need to accept the fact that you are probably hypoglycemic.

5) Parasites

Stool tests done on CFS patients demonstrate that over 80% of the time parasites are present. (See chapter on parasites) [17]

6) Candida Infection (Yeast)

This is another problem that is not easily diagnosed using standard medical tests. Refer to chapter on yeast infections - how to self diagnose this condition.

7) Subclinical Hypothyroidism

Up to 70% of CFS patients have a hypothyroidism problem. That is why I recommend kelp, which is a natural source of iodine, to help replace the deficiency produced by a low functioning thyroid.[18]

8) Low Blood Pressure

This is due to adrenal gland insufficiency and will be explained in greater detail later in this book.

9) Red Blood Cell Damage

CFS patients (over 90%) show red blood cell wall damage upon examination with live cell microscopy.

CHAPTER THREE

Cells - The Key To Life

In order to get to the bottom line of chronic fatigue syndrome, we have to go back to the basic cell. It is at this cell level that Chronic Fatigue Syndrome has a foothold. To return to a higher level of health than Chronic Fatigue Syndrome has allowed you to have, it is necessary to learn all you can about the cell. If you help your cells to return to health, then your whole body will be healthy, since your body is made up of cells. The average human has approximately 100 trillion cells.

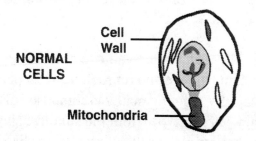

NORMAL CELLS

Cell Wall

Mitochondria

There are four factors that must work together and be in balance in order to promote a healthy body:

1)   Cell environment - your cells are surrounded by fluid (called interstitial fluid). Since most of it is composed of water, it is safe to say that the quality of water that you take in is critical to your cell environment.

2)   Cell communication -Your cells communicate and act in unison partly as a result of transmission between the cells and the brain. If transmission is not clear then the cells do not communicate properly.

3)   Cell exercise - Muscles are made up of cells. Jumping up and down is actually good for the cell and can actually improve the flow of interstitial fluid between the cells. This helps create better circulation, which affects everything else in the cell.

4)   Cell food - In order for the cell to operate, it need nutrients. You are what you eat and what you absorb.

These Four Factors Are Seriously Affected In Chronic Fatigue:

A healthy cell must be able to react to stimuli, maintain a constant balance and reproduce. Most people realise that the majority of living matter is composed of cells. Even though they vary in type, from the smallest single cell organism to the complex multicellular beings like human beings, their basic structure changes little. All cells, for example, are bound by that true cell wall, which in itself surrounds an outer membrane. The contents of a cell, in simple terms, consist of the cytoplasm and the nucleus. There are a few odds and ends hanging around the cytoplasm - they include the mitochondria, some complex carbohydrates and ribosomes. These membranes are all vital to health, of course, but the key to health is the tongue-twisting deoxyribonucleic acid, which scientists around the world have shortened to DNA.

The Free Radical Theory

Through normal metabolism or exposure to pollutants, radiation, and certain medications, oxygen molecules can lose an electron and become unstable particles known as free radicals.

When the free radical theory was first introduced by Doctor Denham Herman in the 1950's, I don't think that he had any idea of the importance of his discovery. Many in the scientific community are now convinced that they have now found a single cause responsible for killer diseases such as heart disease and cancer as well as other ailments such as premature aging and Chronic Fatigue Syndrome.

Dr. Cooper, author of "The Antioxidant Revolution", [19] examines the diseases that are linked by medical research to the insidious operation of free radicals in the body.

I was not at all surprised to discover that it read like the index of a medical encyclopedia. He mentions more than 50 conditions including stroke, asthma, pancreatitis, inflammatory bowel diseases (diverticulitis, ulcerative colitis, peptic ulcers), chronic congestive heart failure, Parkinson's disease, sickle cell disease, leukemia, rheumatoid arthritis, bleeding within the cavity of the brain and high blood pressure. Free radicals have also been implicated in cancer of the lungs, cervix, skin, stomach, prostate, colon and the esophagus.

Free Radicals Set Off Chain Reactions

Seeking to restore balance, a free radical takes an electron from another molecule, creating a new free radical in the process. As each newly-generated free radical looks for a replacement electron, a chain reaction is created.

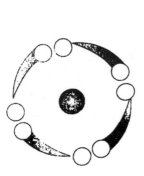

**Normal Oxygen
Atom**

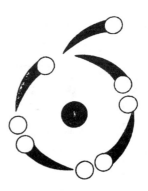

**Electron Loss
Creates Free Radical**

The Hazards Of Oxidation

If this chain of free radical reactions is not broken, it can compromise the integrity of the cell membrane, ultimately damaging the cell.

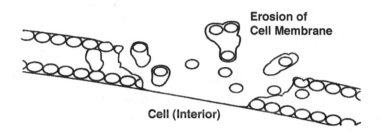

Erosion of Cell Membrane

Cell (Interior)

Antioxidants Neutralize Free Radicals

The molecular structure of antioxidants allows them to give up electrons to free radicals without becoming unstable themselves. This effectively neutralizes the free radicals and breaks the chain of reactions.

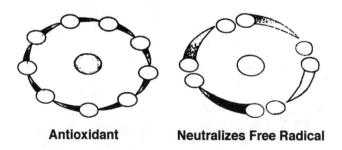

Antioxidant   **Neutralizes Free Radical**

Oxygen - Jekyl and Hyde Syndrome

When I am conducting my seminars, I always like to do an experiment which shows free radical damage. Lemon juice, a mild source of vitamin C antioxidant, is placed on one half of an apple, the other half is left exposed. Within a short period of time, there is a distinct difference between the two halves.

The side that has been protected by the mild antioxidant continues to remain relatively white and unscathed by the elements, whereas, the side that has been left unprotected shrivels up and turns brown very quickly. Although this is an accelerated version of the ravages of free radical damage, it is nonetheless an accurate depiction of what happens to our bodies when we do not protect ourselves. **The villain is oxygen.** This Jekyl and Hyde product of nature, with which we need to live happens to be the very same element that is going to insist that we die.

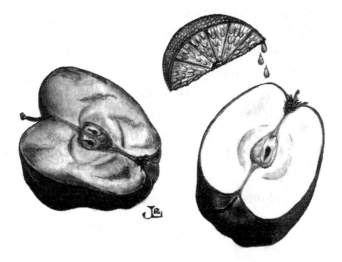

When oxygen is kept in balance we can prevent premature aging of the cells and premature disease which is our ultimate goal. The problem is not so much that oxygen will attack an apple, but what damage this same oxygen, in the form of free radicals, can inflict inside the body. Yet, free radicals are not all bad. When free radicals are kept in balance in the body, they help to detoxify foreign chemicals, fight infection and benefit the mitochrondria of the cell where free radicals release energy.

Keep in mind, however, that outside of this controlled environment, free radicals destroy cellular membranes, enzymes and life itself. Free radicals are an accident looking for a place to occur. Virtually everything useful, is also potentially lethal, but such is life. Controlled free radicals go a long way towards maintaining good health. Many experts now believe that free radicals pose one of the greatest single threat to our public health as we approach the brave new world of the 21st century. [20] Another analogy I like to use in my seminars concerns a person buying an automobile. If, for instance, you go out and buy an 1999 automobile, it is almost guaranteed that by the year 2002 or 2003 you will start to see rust spots and fading paint which are all signs of oxidation to the body of the car. Now, if you take that same vehicle and add a layer of rust proofing on the inner part of the body, you are protecting it from premature aging and thus preserving your investment.

Cell Under Free Radical Attack

It is dangerous, health-wise, for free radicals to tear open the cell wall. Vital cellular chromium can leak into the bloodstream, which in the end has proven to be one of the causes of the onset of adult diabetes and hypoglycemia. Cellular potassium and magnesium can also be lost. Sodium and calcium can get into the cell which has been shown to be the major cause of hypertension. Free radicals are expelling vital ions and chemicals from within the cell and are allowing the sodium, calcium and other contaminants into the cell. Chromium, potassium and magnesium work beautifully in their comfortable environment, inside the safety of the cell wall.

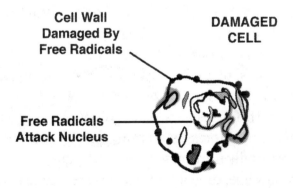

Aging Gracefully

What then makes our health so different? Should we not be willing to make a long-term investment in protecting ourselves against free radical scavengers? Just like our cars will not last forever, we are all one day going to die -

it is inevitable. And yes, we are all going to age, there is no way around this. The point I am trying to make is that there is no reason why we have to age prematurely. Antioxidants, when used properly, will protect and act as a rust proofer for our cells. The cell, as I mentioned earlier, is the basic unit of life. When out of control, free radicals damage the cell wall to such an extent that it is no longer able to prevent the onslaught of free radicals to the mitrochondria which results in conditions such as Chronic Fatigue Syndrome. If not stopped, scavengers can eventually attack the genetic material within the cell (RNA and DNA). At this point, free radicals have become killers, causing these damaged cells to multiply uncontrollably thus resulting in cancer.

Relationship Between Free Radicals and CFS

Oxidation is the loss of electrons, which are those tiny pockets of energy that are in perpetual motion within atoms and molecules.

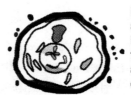

Pycnogenol® antioxidant barrier keeping free radicals away from the cell wall

Living things age, die and decay because they cannot forever control this loss of electrons and the energy contained within them. What would be expected if the rate of energy loss were accelerated? **FATIGUE!!!** This is indeed when a world class sprinter collapses at the finish line and then 5 minutes later he recovers. What would happen if this energy loss was accelerated chronically? **CHRONIC FA-TIGUE!!!** What would happen if the normal free radicals were relentlessly overdriven by allergic triggers (such as mould), chemical sensitivities, antibiotics, pesticides and other pollutants, such as stress, poor dietary habits, junk food, poor physical fitness or even over exercising? Unrelenting chronic fatigue. [21]

Free radical damage deforms cell membranes in CFS patients. Examination of the red blood cells in-patients with CFS (using a high resolution phase contrast microscope) shows deformities of the red cell membrane. [22] There was also a loss of normal elasticity of the cell walls in up to 80% of the cells. Over a period of time the immune system cannot properly do its job of protecting the body against attack from bacteria, viruses and anything else the body normally finds threatening. [23]

ATP

ATP, which stands for adenosine triphoshate, is a high energy substance produced by the mitochondria within our cells. Mitochondria are our little 'Eveready batteries' within our cells. If free radicals caused by nutritional, environmental or lifestyle factors damage the mitochondria within the cell - you guessed it- you have a lack of energy.

↓ ATP = ↓ ENERGY

What Is The Immune System?

The immune system is our body's defence mechanism. It requires exquisite care. One must supply it with the right food, air, water and exercise. Malnutrition damages the immune system more than any other system in the body. Insults from a wide variety of medications, recreational drugs and alcohol, compound the problem. Chronic pain and emotional problems including anxiety, depression and relentless worry also exact their toll on this powerful but delicate system.

A gradual immune decline occurs due to repeated abuse of the sensitive immune apparatus by years of consuming the typical Western high calorie, high fat diet. The use of birth control pills, tranquilizers, exposure to environmental toxins like lead mercury, cadmium, pesticides in fruits and vegetables also contribute to immune decline. Chronic stress also sets the stage but sudden massive stress like death in the family, a divorce or job loss is often the final blow that precipitates a long-term bout of CFS.

While the immune system is still a perplexing and largely unexplained entity, enough is known to give us remarkable insight into the body's amazing ability to protect itself against infection. The immune system is made up of specialized cells. Normally the immune system is able to recognize and respond to millions of different **foreign intruders**, referred to as **antigens. An antigen is anything that triggers an immune response.** The chief players in that response are called white blood cells. There are trillions of white blood cells in the body at any one time. The majority of them are stored in such areas as the spleen and lymph nodes. There are **many different classes of white blood cells**. The most notable of these are divided into **three groups**, depending on the function that they serve. These are the **T-cells, B-cells and the macrophages.**

The T-Cell

When a virus enters the body it is the circulating T-cell that recognizes it as a foreign antigen. The T-cell is one of the most important aspects of the immune system. When a T-cell comes into contact with this antigen, it calls for reinforcements by releasing chemical signals into the blood stream. Another important, perhaps crucial, type of T-cell is called the "Natural Killer" (NK) cell. NK cells function as scavengers in the immune system. In CFS and Fibromyalgia sufferers the NK cells do not function properly.

The B-Cell

The main function of B-cells is to produce deadly proteins called antibodies. B-cells produce specific antibodies that destroy specific viruses. This precise response serves two purposes: 1) It ensures that these powerful antibodies will attack only foreign invaders and not cells of the body. 2) It also serves as a type of memory system, allowing the immune system to remember a specific infectious agent.

When the infection is over, the immune system retains these specific antibodies used against the invaders. The next time the intruders will have a harder time attacking. One B-cell would not be able to produce enough antibodies to handle thousands of viruses. It needs help from a third type of white blood cell called macrophages.

Macrophages

Macrophages, the largest of the white blood cells, have many functions. One of the most important duties that the macrophage performs is that these cells destroy viruses by swallowing and engulfing them. The macrophages in the CFS and Fibromyalgia person are not able to perform their proper task because of extensive free radical damage over a period of time.

The immune system can be explained in simple terms. If a person goes boating and the motor hits a rock, the boat would stop running. Two different makes of motors might react in different ways, depending on the workmanship and sturdiness of the model of the motor. The human system, of course, is far more complex than the motor of a boat, but, at the same time incredibly adaptable. The adaptability allows the immune system to defend against many types of invaders: bacteria, viruses and fungi. If the delicate system is sufficiently disturbed, the immune system can stop working, in differing degrees from person to person. This depends on the strength of the immune system before the invasion, or the immune system can even attack the body itself. When the immune system becomes confused and attacks the body, an "autoimmune disease" can develop. When a person develops CFS, the checks and balances within the healthy immune system are disrupted. The cells don't communicate properly with each other, and they don't know how to respond appropriately to invaders.

THE CANCER CONNECTION - Good Cells Gone Bad

Cancer is a disorder characterized by a weak immune system and uncontrolled multiplying of cells due to free radical damage over a long period of time. [24] Guess what the first step to cancer is and the bottom-line of Chronic Fatigue Syndrome? A weak immune system and uncontrolled multiplying of cells because of free radical damage over a long period of time! Cancer cells are continually attacking our bodies each day. Even if we ate the best nutritional diet possible, the very digestive process that your body uses to breakdown food produces chemical by-products called "free radicals". There are also other metabolic functions in our body that produce "free radicals". Our healthy cells are constantly being attacked by these free radicals by trying to change our DNA and thus forming cancer cells. When this happens, our immune system is consistently not "up to snuff". These cancerous cells multiply and a tumor will grow inside of you. [25]

15 Years - 500 Cases

Now that I have been tracking Chronic Fatigue for almost 15 years, let me issue a warning. A woman who has Chronic Fatigue Syndrome becomes nearly twice as likely to develop breast or colon cancer than the average female. Folks, Chronic Fatigue, if not treated properly, can literally kill!! I now call CFS the pre - cancer disease. [26]

Why CFS Can Lead To Cancer

Even though most research on cancer today involves genes - in my opinion it is almost a complete waste of time and money. There are some factors that are so obvious that we are missing them right under our noses. A woman's immune system becomes compromised because of stress, heavy workload, dietary and environmental factors and even reasons such as prolonged antibiotic use, and the birth control pill. Her body's defence mechanism becomes a sitting duct for a collapse. Therefore, a woman stands very little chance to fight cancer actively in her body. Unfortunately, cancer cells can multiply for several months or years without really showing any symptoms other than perhaps fatigue.

Women Are Canaries

I come from a mining town in Northern Ontario, Canada. Often stories were told of miners who would take canaries with them underground. Canaries had very small body systems and if there were any toxic gas leaks in the mine they would die. When this happened the miners knew to get out of the mine quickly in order to save their own lives. Women have become the modern day canaries. Their body systems are more fragile for the several reasons that we have already explained. Women are dying like flies from all sorts of cancer. Now if one out of seven women is going to get breast cancer then you ladies with Chronic Fatigue Syndrome and Fibromyalgia must be even more cautious.

BOTTOM LINE

Here's what we have to do to prevent cancer:

• Cut down on meat and dairy products.
• Take a daily dose of antioxidants such as Pycnogenol®
  and beta-carotene.
• Drink plenty of pure filtered water.
• Increase daily intake of fruits and vegetables.
• Stop smoking and reduce as much exposure
  as possible to second hand smoke.
• Be careful in the sun.
• Exercise regularly - at least 5 times per week.
• Increase fiber in the diet.
• Cut down on caffeine.
• Have a good positive mental outlook - start your day by
  praying and reading the Bible for guidance and comfort
  in this crazy world.
• It is especially important for women - make sure that you
  remain yeast and parasite free.

CHAPTER FOUR

The Stress Connection

Stress is one of the leading causes of immune system depression.

External Stress

This is how we deal with outside stress. A lot of this outside stress is how we perceive the world around us. It is what we think is happening to us and our interpretation of our circumstances. External stresses entail:

- Threats to safety
- Psychological triggers (excitement, anger, frustration, irritation, worry)
- Challenges
- Confrontations
- Hardships

Internal Stress

This is stress that is initiated from the inside. Internal stresses includes:

- Illness and disease process
- Depression
- Pain
- Discomfort

Internal stress, such as repeated infections, long-term antibiotic use or continuous worry and anxiety, can reduce the response of the immune system in Chronic Fatigue Syndrome. External stress, such as trauma from a car accident or constant pain can lead to fibromyalgia.

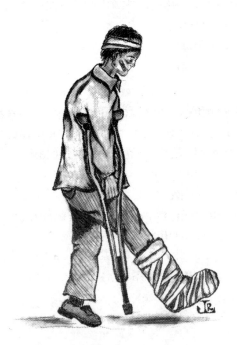

All of these stressors cause the brain to send messages to two areas of the body. The first to the pituitary gland, and the second message is to the brain stem and spinal cord, which alerts many parts of the body, including the adrenal glands. There are signals sent out that cause the release of chemicals and hormones. Two of these hormones from the adrenal gland, adrenaline and noradrenaline, cause the "fight or flight" mechanism. This hormone allows our body to physically be prepared to attack the source of stress or to run from it. Adrenaline and noradrenaline, when released into the bloodstream, stimulate the heart, raise blood pressure, send glucose to muscles and increases cholesterol. In a normal response, adrenaline can give a person a feeling of well-being, excitement or euphoria and a reduced need to sleep. The adrenal gland also excretes hormones, like cortisol and cortisone, which help fight pain and inflammation, increases blood sugar, frees fatty acids, and increases muscle tension. [27]

Continually Revved Up Body

When you run a motor for a period of time it helps clear out carbon and other unwanted things that have built up. If that motor is left running for a period of long time, the reverse happens and carbon deposits collect on the valves. It then wears out much faster. This is a good example of what constant stress, like-Chronic Fatigue, does to our bodies. Wear it out! Chronic Fatigue is an internal stress and your body cannot turn it off. This is the first reason why CFS patients suffer from debilitating fatigue, allergies, sleep disorders, sweet cravings, and cognitive problems. You cannot live in this constant crisis state and not pay for it physically. The body reaps what it sows.

Since the action of stress has lowered the immune system, other systems in our body fail to do their job. As a result, sufferers of Chronic Fatigue most likely are also sufferers of adrenal gland mysfunction, hypoclycemia, hypothyroidism, altered brain wave patterns, yeast infections and allergies. An imbalance in estrogen and progesterone in women, can cause the symptoms related to PMS or menopause.

The next chapter on adrenal gland mysfunction is one of the results of a continually stressed body and explores the complex causes and far reaching effects on our cells and ultimately our total body performance. This gives us a little more insight into such a complex illness. No wonder a person with Chronic Fatigue Syndrome feel sick and tired all of the time.

The Adrenal-Hypothalamus Gland Connection

Dr. Jacob Teitelbaum MD postulates in his excellent book, " From Fatigued to Fantastic", [28] that the Hypothalamus is adversely affected in people suffering from CFS. The reason that this happens is unclear. I suggest that after a person's immune system is compromised they become susceptible to a viral type infection. Viruses such as Mono, Epstein Barr or others can only attack a system that is previously weakened. I believe the virus invasion or even mycotoxins can cause the brain to swell and subsequently the hypothalamus gland becomes affected.

Hypothalamus Gland

The hypothalamus gland, which is located at the base of the brain, is perhaps the most important gland in the whole body. This gland, in reality, regulates all other glands. For example, if the hypothalamus is suppressed, due to brain swelling, it can lead to problems with the pineal, thyroid, pituitary and the adrenal glands.

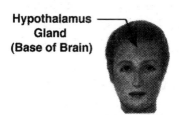

Hypothalamus
Gland
(Base of Brain)

In the next several chapters we will discuss the dysfunction of the adrenal gland, which has a great affect on CFS patients who suffer from hypoglycemia, asthma, allergies and a host of other symptoms. Keep in mind that the adrenal gland only becomes affected when the hypothalamus gland is suppressed.

Adrenal Gland

The adrenal glands curve over the top of each kidney in the abdomen. They secrete key stress hormones such as cortisol, DHEA, and adrenaline. In chronic fatigue sufferers these hormones are often at abnormal levels which is called the continual stress response. These hormones can influence a number of body functions, from immune response to the kind of sleep we get at night.

With the abnormal secretions of hormones, fatigue and muscle pain may result.

Stressors That Tax The Adrenal Gland Are:

- Physical trauma
- Poor Diet
- Lack of Sleep
- Emotional Trauma
- Prescription Drugs
- Chemical Toxins
- Excessive Exercise
- Infections
- Anxiety
- Depression
- Pregnancy

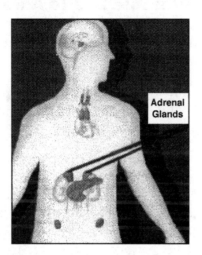

The signs and symptoms of overtaxed adrenal glands are :

- Fatigue
- Irritability
- Inability to concentrate
- Frustration
- Insomnia
- Sweet cravings
- Allergies
- Nervousness
- Depression
- Weakness, light headedness
- Pre-menstrual tension
- Headaches

Chronic Fatigue Syndrome And Low Blood Pressure Due To Adrenal Insufficiency

Researchers at Johns Hopkins Children's Centre reported a link between hypotension (low blood pressure) and symptoms of CFS. [29] In one study, 4 of 7 adolescents between the ages of 12 and 16, had prompt improvement in their chronic fatigue when hypotension was treated with Atenolol or Disopyramide for light-headedness. The adrenal glands work to control blood pressure by secreting cortisone and adrenaline. Cortisone triggers sodium water retention throughout the body while adrenaline causes constriction of the arteries. Adrenal insufficiency or exhaustion due to excessive physical, chemical and/or emotional stress (as is common with Chronic Fatigue Syndrome) causes blood vessel walls to become loose and flaccid. Light-headedness or faintness may be experienced when standing quickly, due to a drop in blood pressure and a delayed blood flow to the brain. This is a common problem for CFS patients. Many members of the natural food and dietary supplement industry are aware of the connection between diet and adrenal exhaustion. Over consumption of refined carbohydrates has an adverse effect on blood sugar controlling mechanisms and places stress on the adrenals to compensate for low blood sugar. Caffeine and other stimulants force the adrenals to work harder, eventually depleting them. These substances must be avoided to allow exhausted adrenals to recuperate. Foods with a high nutrient density along with appropriate supplements nourish and energize the glands, not deplete them. Nutrients that have special importance to the adrenal glands are the B vitamins (particularly pantothenic acid), vitamin C, magnesium, potassium, tyrosine, and phenylanoline. Both tyrosine and phenylanoline are converted into thyroid and adrenal hormones. One of the most prominent signs of adrenal gland insufficiency is chronic fatigue. As a response to stress, the adrenal glands produce DHEA and cortisol. Both hormones have predictable effects on body chemistry. In health, the ratio of the two is optimal. The hypothalamus and the pituitary gland, both in the brain, are sensitive to the amount of cortisol circulating in the blood. When cortisol reaches a certain level, the hypothalamus and pituitary levels are properly regulated. However, certain factors may overload this system. During chronic stress, excessive cortisol is often produced. Moreover, the hypothalamus and pituitary gland may grow less sensitive to the changes and may not turn off production of cortisol as they should. When this happens, a series of problems may occur, such as decreased immune system function, altered blood sugar regulation, fat accumulation and changes in behaviour. If chronic stress persists, more cortisol is produced, but less DHEA. As the amount of cortisol becomes higher, while DHEA becomes lower, the adverse health consequences grow. Meanwhile, excessive epinephrine (or adrenaline) is produced which has its own set of adverse consequences. The adrenal glands produce their array of hormones in a complex symphony that is orchestrated by two structures in the brain, the hypothalamus and the pituitary gland. When stress and poor nutrition lead to altered hormone levels, imbalance in endocrine function can lead to substantial fatigue. The only road back appears to be stress management coupled with appropriate biochemical therapy.

No wonder a person with Chronic Fatigue Syndrome feels sick and fatigued all of the time.

The Hypoglycemic Connection

Hypoglycemia and Chronic Fatigue go hand in hand. I have rarely treated anyone with CFS who is not suffering from hypoglycemia. Since the cells are so damaged throughout the body, from continual stress like allergies, adrenal problems, thyroid dysfunction and depression, what should be inside the cell has leaked out (chromium), and what is outside the cell has been absorbed in.

Hypoglycemia simply means low blood sugar. The average American ingests 134 pounds of sugar per year. The body cannot handle the concentrated sugars that often make up a large part of our diet. The pancreas overreacts by producing too much insulin. This depletes the blood sugar and causes the body to cry out for more food. Usually the wrong food choice is made and a viscous circle is started. The brain and central nervous system derive their support from adequate supplies of blood sugar. Low blood sugar has most of its effect on the function of the brain and nervous symptoms. [30] Can you recognise yourself in this pattern of hypoglycemia?

1) Excessive intake of refined carbohydrates

2) Rapid rise of blood sugar

3) Excessive production of insulin by the pancreas

4) Rapid decline in blood sugar due to excess insulin

5) Adrenal gland converts glycogen to sugar for emergency

6) Adrenal glands do not respond properly and don't know when to quit

7) Body needs sugar fast!

8) Wrong food with a high sugar content ingested

9) Blood sugar rises rapidly and cycle starts all over again

10) Repetition of this vicious circle many times a day

The hypoglycemic person eats sugar, but after inges-tion the blood sugar level rises and then quickly bottoms out because the pancreas cannot handle the concentrated sugar. The body cries out for more food, but the wrong kind is eaten and the vicious circle starts over again.

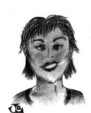
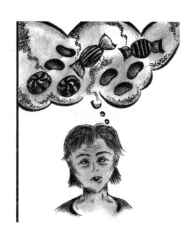

Symptoms of Hypoglycemia

Hypoglycemic episodes can minic almost every neurologic and psychiatric disorder. The most common symptoms of hypoglycemia are:

→   Fatigue, Exhaustion, Headaches

→   Irritability, Insomnia, Overactivity in Children, Behavorial Problems, Short Temper

→   Eczema, Hives, Sinusitis

→   Nervousness, Anxiety, Depression, Crying Spells, Fearfulness, Personality Changes

→   Inability to Concentrate, Forgetfulness, Fog Over the Brain, Prolonged Sleepiness

→   Palpitations and Irregular Heartbeat

→ Feelings of Faintness, Dizziness, Tremors, Cold
   Sweats, Water Retention

→ Inner Trembling, Shortness of Breath, Asthma, Hay
   Fever

→ Digestive Disorders- Colitis, Diarrhea, Stomach Pain

→ Blurred Vision, Cold Extremities
→ Craving for Sweets, Alcohol, Coffee, or Cola

→ Uncontrollable Weight Gain

→ Seizures, Convulsions

Hypoglycemic Blood Sugar Test

The normal six hour reading should be within five
percent of the fasting level. No point should fall below the
baseline. The one hour level should rise at least 50% above
the fasting level. In a test for hypoglycemia 100 grams of
sugar (glucose) is ingested after a fast of twelve hours. A
blood test is taken just before the glucose is ingested and
then again each hour for six hours. In the following charts
0 is used as the baseline for the six hour blood test. The
circumstances for the test are ideal and controlled and not
those of everyday life. A patient may only show borderline
hypoglycemic here, but with the everyday stress of life there
is added strain on the adrenal glands and the blood sugar
drop is more drastic.

Normal Blood Sugar Chart

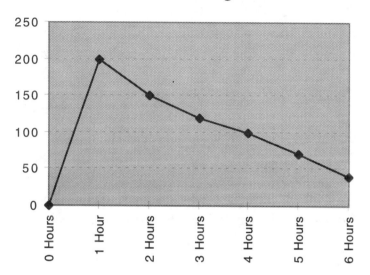

Hypoglycemic Blood Sugar Chart

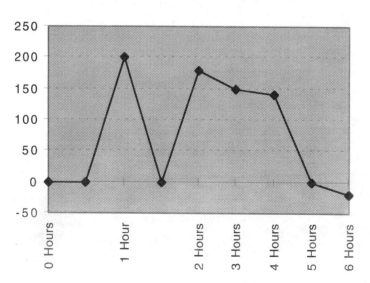

Hypoglycemic Blood Sugar Curve

This is the result of only a mild hypoglycemic. In more severe cases the three hour blood sugar is already below the 0 baseline. There is also the case scenario where the blood sugar dips only below the 0 baseline by only one or two points. Here the blood sugar dips below the 0 baseline. The five hour blood sugar is -10 and the six hour is -20. At this point the person is feeling all the symptoms of hypoglycemia and the viscous circle is started. To further complicate things it should be noted that the symptoms of hypoglycemia can be mimicked by Candida ablicans overgrowth in the stomach, or by food allergies. Cancer and yeast also loves and grows on sugar.

No wonder a person with Chronic Fatigue Syndrome feels sick and fatigued all of the time.

The Allergy Connection

I believe that there are the rare Chronic Fatigue Syndrome sufferers who do not suffer from allergies. An allergy is an unfavourable immune system reaction to a substance, food or inhaled (environmental), that most people find harmless. A food allergy is the immune system's reaction to a certain food, when the body creates IgE antibodies to that food. When these IgE antibodies react with the food, histamine and other chemicals (called mediators) are released from various cells within the body. Eight foods cause 90% of all the food reactions. They are milk, egg, wheat, peanut, soy, tree nuts, fish, and shellfish. Dr. Leon Chaitow, N.D., D.O., of London, England, has been researching allergies for a number of years and has found that a number of factors negatively impact the immune system. These factors include toxic burden due to pollution in all its forms. [31]

Hidden or "Masked" Food Allergies

In masked food allergies, the body compensates with an addiction to the offending food. People are allergic to the ingested food, but, the body craves it. The very food we crave makes us sick. The best way to experiment, to see if you have food allergies, is to eliminate something that you find that you eat every day. This might be peanut butter, or eggs. Do not eat them for a period of three weeks. This is when all of the substance will be out of your system. After this time period, sit down and eat whatever you have been abstaining from. Allergic symptoms can begin within minutes to one hour after ingesting the food.

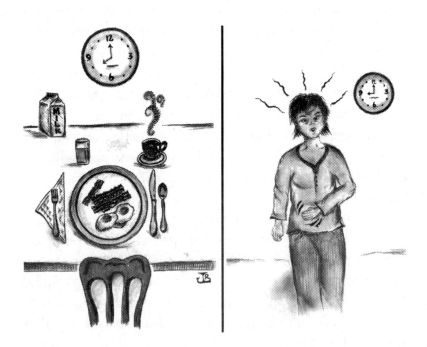

Checklist of Allergic Symptoms In Body Systems

Gastrointestinal System

Allergies can provoke gastrointestinal discomforts like heartburn, indigestion, bloating, passing gas, abdominal pain, cramps, diarrhea, and constipation. [32] One of the reasons that a sufferer with chronic fatigue syndrome puts on weight is because of food allergies. The easiest thing for the body to do when it comes in contact with a food that it is allergic to, is store it as fat. Most of these sufferers are unaware that they even have food allergies. If you feel that you have to lie down after you have eaten a meal to digest it, or if you suffer from spastic colon and irritable bowel syndrome maybe you should look into food allergies. The inappropriate use of antibiotics could be the cause of the development of food allergies. A large percentage of chronic fatigue patients have histories of recurrent antibiotic treatment as children and adults.

Respiratory System

Allergies can also affect the **respiratory** system in the form of a runny nose, sneezing, cough or wheeze, night cough, asthma, shortness of breath, bronchitis and emphysema.

How Food Allergies Affects The Cardiovascular System

Rapid heartbeat, palpitations, skipped heartbeats, chest pain, flushing, chills, hot flashes, night sweats, high or low blood pressure can all be related to other illnesses. Medication may be prescribed that are specifically for these illnesses, and after a period of time, there is no noticeable improvement, and other medications are prescribed. You are now dealing with all of the side effects from these drugs, and the underlying problem, which still has not been resolved.

Miscellaneous Conditions Of Food Allergies

Anemia, addictions (alcohol, foods, drugs), tiredness, uterine fibroids, fibrocystic breast disease, cancer, and autoimmune disease are just a few of the areas that are being researched in relation to allergies. The eyes can also be affected. Eye pain, itching, sensitivity to light, blurred vision, puffy lids, allergic black eyes, red, bloodshot eyes and constant blinking.

Environmental Allergies

Many chronic illnesses today are the result of lifestyle habits and /or exposure to a variety of substances found in the places that we live, work, and in the food we eat. The people with environmental allergies can present multisystemic disorders. The physical and mental symptoms can leave the sufferer in a state of misery for years on end. To add insult to injury these symptoms are dismissed and treated as psychosomatic. The more symptoms a patient accumulates, the less likely the doctor will take their complaints legitimately. There can be physical and psychological signs and symptoms to a patient's environmental exposure at home, work or school, different seasons or effects of diet. Here are some symptoms:

→   hyper after lunch or bulky supper (diet, allergies)

→   tired and sleepy 30 minutes after a meal (diet, allergies, hypoglycemia)

→   recurrent upper respiratory, ear infections (diet, allergies)

→   recurrent urinary problems (diet, candida)

→   depression (diet, mold or chemical exposure)

→   irritation of eyes, throat, breathing problems, lack of concentration, tiredness after renovation, new carpets, new furniture etc. (chemical exposure)

The Yeast Connection (Candida Albicans)

Anyone who suffers from Chronic Fatigue Syndrome, most likely suffers from a Candidia infection. [33] What is Candida? Candida is the name that is given to different species of yeasts. One of the most common unfriendly yeast organisms in our body is Candida Albicans. Normally it is kept in balance by friendly bacteria but when the balance is upset, the Candida multiplies. As its numbers grow, the normally non-invasive yeast changes to a fungus-like microbe and releases toxins into the blood stream, which produces the debilitating effects of Candida infection. If you are eating improperly, ingesting large amounts of sugar, taking antibiotics, or changing your body chemistry with birth control pills, you are providing the perfect environment for yeast to multiply uncontrollably. It is common knowledge that antibiotics, especially over a period of time or with repeated use, will eliminate much of the normal microbes of the gastrointestinal tract. As a result of the elimination of the normal flora defence mechanism, the yeast is allowed to grow excessively in the gut. In this day and age when physicians are increasingly and liberally prescribing oral antibiotics, intestinal Candida proliferation is becoming an increasing problem.

Have You Ever Wondered Why So Many People Recently Seem To Be Suffering From Chronic Fatigue Syndrome Along With Irritable Bowel Syndrome?

It is now known that the whole digestive tract is coated with a thin layer of living bacteria. This "friendly bacteria" actually forms a vital structure known as "anaerobic paste" which creates a protective barrier. This barrier can be destroyed by antibiotics, junk food diets, drug or alcohol and mercury amalgam fillings. This barrier keeps the proper things in the intestinal tract and rids the intestines of the wrong things. Candida has been a suspect in playing a part in creating what is called an unfavorable increase in intestinal permeability. [34] This simply means that the contents of the gut contain toxic materials and normally the body puts up a barrier so that these toxins do not enter the blood stream. However, with a "leaky gut" undigested macromolecule, food particles and toxins are allowed to pass directly into the body's bloodstream through penetrations in the intestinal wall, creating a host of problems. Diseases that have been associated with "leaky gut" are

Chron's disease, irritable bowel syndrome, diarrhea, cholera, hepatitis, cystic fibrosis, chemical sensitivities, environmental illnesses, hyperactivity, inflammatory bowel disease and alcoholism.

Toxic "Leaky Gut"

Candida has been found to produce 79 different toxins, which creates havoc with the immune system. A person is told that they have become environmentally sensitive and has allergic reactions to various "harmless" inhalants in the environment, as well as various foods. These reactions do not create typical allergic symptoms. Because of the strain on the immune system to break down these undigested molecules, the body's ability to defend against Candida may be further weakened, creating a cycle. These particles may also pass through the blood/brain barrier, and produce other mental symptoms that may create a misdiagnosis of neurotic disorder. Research is currently being done at the National Institute for Health into the Candida cycle. The Candida Syndrome is a series of vague, sometimes seemingly unrelated symptoms. The person may even be referred to a psychiatrist for their "neurotic condition" and the failure of modern science to find a physiological diagnosis. Routine blood tests usually never reveal anything unusual.

Symptoms Of Candida Albicans Infection

→ **Nervous System** - depression or manic depression, attacks of anxiety or crying, sudden mood swings, lack of concentration, drowsiness, poor memory, headaches, light headedness, insomnia, fatigue, or feeling of being drained.

→ **Digestive System**- abdominal bloating, pain and gas, indigestion, heartburn, constipation, diarrhea, gastritis, sensitivity to milk, wheat, corn, or other common foods.

→ **Urinary/Vaginal Area**- Recurrent bladder infections, burning or urgent urinations, cystitis, vaginal burning or itching, menstrual cramping.

→ **Musculoskeletal System**- muscle and/or joint swelling and pain, muscle weakness, cold hands and feet, or low body temperature.

→ **Mouth and Throat**- bleeding gums, dry mouth and tongue, cracked tongue, thrush, white patches in the mouth, bad breath, sore throat, laryngitis, cough or recurrent bronchitis, pain or tightness in chest, wheezing or shortness of breath.

→ **Skin**- hives, athlete's foot, fungus infection of the nails, jock itch, psoriasis, or chronic skin rashes.

No wonder a person with Chronic Fatigue Syndrome feels sick and fatigued all of the time.

C H A P T E R   N I N E

The Parasite Connection

What Is A Parasite?

The Chronic Fatigue Sufferer is particularly at risk for the invasion of parasites because of a depleted immune system and a stifled body defence mechanism. [35] It is not difficult for the parasites to find a friendly environment in the intestines. A parasite is any organism, whether a single cell or a eight meter long tapeworm, that lives invasively in your body and produces toxins from its body secretions.

How is this possible in this day and age? Well, have you **played with a cat or dog recently?** Parasites and worms thrive on animals. **Have you shared somebody else's pop can? or even shook someone's hand lately?** Ever **nibbled at the supermarket on strawberries or**

grapes or even eaten fruit that has not been washed properly? Do you **eat fast food often?** When was the last time you drank **tap water?** How about the **bacon** you had for breakfast this morning, or the **roast beef** you had for supper last night?

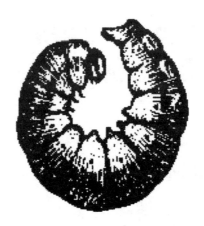

Parasites are a major threat to your health. They reproduce quickly and can cause **allergies** by secreting toxins and wastes into your system. Miscroscopic parasites can get into your joints and eat the linings of the bone. This can lead to **arthritic** tendencies. Parasites cause **malnutrition** by stealing vital nutrients from the intestinal tract, blood and even directly from the cells. The **parasites eat the nutrients even before you do!!** They take the best nutrients, and you are left with the scraps and leftovers. This renders your cells incapable of repairing themselves and ultimately **destroying your health.** Parasites eat human bodies and can live off the host (your body) for years. If you are a person who craves sugar, you may have a sugar-loving parasite.

Signs Of Parasites In Your Body

Allergies gas and bloating, eating more than normal but still feeling hungry, chronic fatigue syndrome, grinding teeth, irritable bowel syndrome, nervousness, constipation, diarrhea, unclear thinking, joint and muscle pain, sleep disturbances, weight gain or weight loss.

What Do You Do To Rid Yourself Of Parasites?

• Whether you think you have parasites or not it is always wise to do a colon/parasitic cleanse a couple times a year. If you have symptoms of disease showing up it is even more imperative.

• Build up your immune system by taking supplements, vitamins and improve your diet

• Exercise regularly and drink 8-10 glasses of distilled or spring water a day.

• Increase your fiber intake - the average person gets 14.5 grams of fiber a day. This is half of what is necessary in a daily diet.

• Don't eat raw fish and cook your beef until it is well done and there is no red showing.

•If you are a camper don't drink from the stream or river.

• Always wash your hands after working in the garden, since soil can contain parasites, and after using the washroom.

• Pets are carriers of parasites and worms so deworm them regularly and don't sleep near your pet.

Over 1,000 species of parasites can live in our bodies, but tests are available for only 40 to 50 types. Doctors are only testing for about 5% of the parasites and missing 80%. **This brings the clinically found parasites down to 1%.** When the immune system becomes weakened, our bodies become susceptible to infections of other kinds. [36]

The parasites nest, feed and lay eggs in our colon. Over time a layer of refuse coats the colon and becomes thicker and thicker. This is uneliminated fecal matter. The colon is still trying to draw nutrients from the matter that is passing through it, but, with the layer of compacted, toxic fecal matter, guess what gets soaked up with the nutrients?- **TOXINS!!** You are poisoning yourself every time you eat!

The Depression Connection - You're Not Alone

One of the symptoms of CFS is depression. <u>But remember depression only comes after the onset of CFS.</u> Hey!! Wouldn't anybody be depressed if they had a hard time even getting out of bed. In literally hundreds of radio and TV interviews, I'm always asked the question - "What does Chronic Fatigue feel like?". I remind the audiences about the last time they had suffered the flu. Then I ask them this: "How would they like to have the flu that never goes away?" Well that is what Chronic Fatigue feels like - <u>The flu that never goes away.</u> No wonder a person that has CFS is depressed. There are still dinosaur doctors out there that think CFS's major cause is depression. These doctors need to realise that this wrong diagnosis has severely abused and maligned literally thousands of women and men in North America.

Once when I was being interviewed on Wisconsin public radio concerning CFS, a medical doctor called on the open line show. He said that everything that I said was interesting, but really CFS was nothing more than mass hysteria. He went on to mention that women were really only depressed and a simple treatment of antidepressants was the cure. Boy! Did I have fun with him! I reminded him that there were hundreds of medical papers on CFS and if he would only keep up on his reading, he would not be so ignorant. However, my rebuke of him was actually quite tame compared to the onslaught of the listeners who phoned the show. Several women, including nurses and other professionals, called and blasted this doctor for his ignorance. But, these same callers mentioned that they were used to receiving this type of abuse by their attending physicians. Doctors, it is time to wake up and smell the coffee. CFS is real and in epidemic proportion today. Taking antidepressants is not the answer!

Depression always comes *__after__* the onset of CFS. Depressive illnesses make you *feel exhausted, worthless, helpless, and hopeless.* To be able to cry would be a relief, but there is an *inability to let these emotions out, especially in tears.* Such *negative thoughts and feelings* make some people feel like giving up. These negative views are part of the depression and typically do not accurately reflect your situation.

There is one important factor that should be taken into account before treating the depression. Recent studies and reports by the U.S. Department of Health and Human

Services show that between *12 and 36 percent of the average psychiatrist's patients are being treated for mental disorders they do not have.* [37] [38]

Change The Name

I really believe that Chronic Fatigue Syndrome ought to have a name change. You know why? Just the mention of the name "Chronic Fatigue Syndrome" seems to trivialize this disorder. People, I think tend to minimize the horrendous effects of Chronic Fatigue Syndrome because of its name. Insurance companies, employers and even doctors often have never taken this syndrome seriously because of the name. I know in Canada and the U.K., the name M.E. or Myalgia Encephalomyletitis (brain swelling) was gaining popularity a few years ago. I know that I would be a big supporter for a name change.

PART 2

The Solution:

Six Weeks To Better Health

Help For The Chronic Fatigue Sufferer

The first part of this book was formulated to give you vital information concerning CFS. I have always been a firm believer that information provides choices. Hopefully now you understand that CFS attacks every organ in your body. What you are about to read in the next section is the solution to Chronic Fatigue Syndrome. I want you to know that we have several hundred documented cases of people with CFS who are following our recommended program and are now living fruitful lives once again. There is hope!!! The first step is to get you to understand your condition. Now if you will follow our program you are going to get results. You will start to see a major improvement in 6 weeks. Don't get discouraged, your body's cells are quite sick and they are in a pre-cancer state.

6 Weeks

There is no real magic to the actual number of 6 weeks, just good old-fashioned common sense. In my experience, while treating literally thousands of patients over 25 years, I've come to some simple observations.

1) It takes 21 days to form a habit
2) It takes another 21 days to enforce that habit

Therefore the 6 weeks solution to CFS comes from my experience with human nature. Friend, if you have Chronic Fatigue Syndrome you need a lifestyle change.

There are four areas that I want to change in your life over the next 6 weeks.

1)   I want to change your mind
2)   I want to change your diet
3)   I want to change your supplement intake
4)   I want to change your exercise philosophy

Changing Your Mind

Attitude

Why do we put such importance on attitude? Well, in my 25 years of practice I've literally known hundreds of patients that, without even knowing it, had no real desire to get better. Let me explain. Patients' sickness sometimes becomes their security blanket. I have known patients who because of their personal problems never really wanted to get healthy. These people were often having marrital problems or other relationship disorders that were not easily solved. Therefore a disorder that they were experiencing became chronic because getting better would have meant they would have to face or solve their personal problem. Sometimes feeling sorry for themselves was the only way that they could cope. Another example is that some of my patients perhaps subconsciously realised that if they got better then they would no longer be the center of attention.

A rotten marriage or other difficulties at home have an enormous impact on the attitude that one might have in helping to solve CFS. So, once again attitude is most important and is involved in the 1st D in my 3D plan for getting better.

OVERALL PHILOSOPHY - The 3 D's

Desire

Getting better from CFS necessitates a complete desire to recover. I can bring you to the water, but I can't make you drink. How bad do you want to get better? Desire involves the mind. You must want this problem solved. You must see yourself getting better.

Determination

Determination involves the heart. I know a lot of alcoholics who have the desire to quit drinking. After they drink they feel sorry for what they have done. But you see they are not really determined at this point. In their head, like smokers wanting to quit, they say "I wish I could quit". Determination brings them to the next level. Now they are saying, "I am going to get better". 1) You must have a desire to get better. 2) You must be determined to get better. Be determined that in the next six weeks if you have a bad day (and you will) **DON'T GIVE UP.** Don't let friends (negative ones) or family discourage you. Take one day at a time, and be faithful to the plan. The next six weeks will literally change your body's cells. You will start to recover and your immune system will start to function again.

Discipline

Desire involves the mind. Determination involves the heart and discipline involves the body. Over the next six weeks we are asking you to discipline your body. If we ask you to eliminate something from your diet or add supplements, then be faithful and disciplined. Your body cells are counting on you. By the way, only you as a sufferer of CFS know how difficult it is, especially on bad days, to even think, let alone act. But, discipline will go a long ways towards recovery.

Are You Ready?

Maybe start with a prayer, asking the Lord to help. I don't believe in coincidences and therefore, you are not reading this book by chance. Ask God to help you stick to the plan and give you wisdom to understand your disease.

Optimism

In his book "Who Gets Sick?" medical writer Blair Justice begins a section with the definition of a pessimist. He writes: "A pessimist is someone who, when confronted with two unpleasant alternatives, selects both". Do not limit your body's ability to get better. A positive attitude or healthy determination and discipline will go a long way to help you recover. Now read on.

Five Steps To Changing Your Diet

1) Cut Down On Your Fat Intake

Be informed and learn all about the different fats (which ones are bad for you and which ones are essential for optimum body functions). Fat is a necessary part of a healthy diet. Not all fats are bad for you. Unfortunately, not many know how to separate the good from the bad. Refined fats are comparable to refined sugar because they are both empty calories. Fats perform vital functions in our body, they:

1)   Cushion and protect our organs.

2)   Serve as building blocks for cell membranes and certain hormones that govern numerous body functions.

3)   Are necessary for the absorption of the fat soluble vitamins A, D, E and K. Too little dietary fat can cause malfunction in the immune and gastrointestinal systems, not to mention the eyes, skin, bones and teeth which these vitamins protect.

THE GOOD

Monosaturated fats are the good guys. These are the ones that keep a balance between the "good" cholesterol (yes, there is actually good cholesterol) HDL or High- Density Lipoprotein and the "bad" cholesterol- LDL or Low-Density Lipoprotein. Olive oil, peanut, almonds, pecans, sesame, canola and avocado are the superior of the oils.

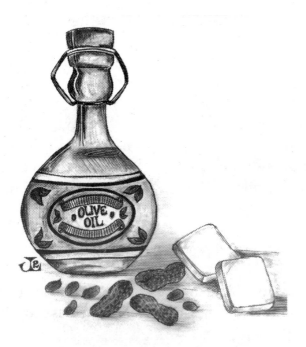

THE BAD

Polyunsaturated fats lower the level of cholesterol, but they also lower the "good" cholesterol- HDL- the one that you want to have lots of. Polyunsaturateds are the most prevalent in packaged products, because they are the most economical. They are found in small amounts in almost all plant foods and in high amounts in most vegetable oils and cold water fish.

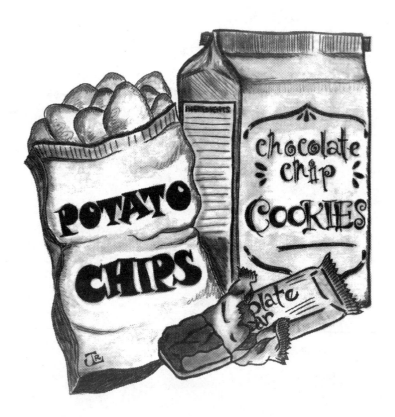

THE UGLY

Saturated fats are the most potent elevators of blood cholesterol. These are the fats that are responsible for blood sludge or artery clogging. Saturated fats are derived from any animal product, cheese, butter, shortening, beef, coconut and full fat dairy products. Chicken, turkey and fish have the least amount of saturated fats.

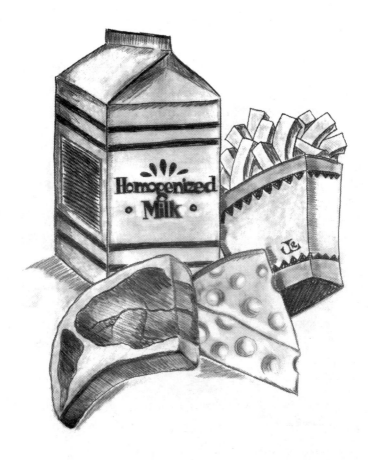

Helpful Ways To Decrease Fat In Your Diet

• Drink more water to control your appetite

• Eat more fiber in place of fat. More fiber gives you the feeling of fullness

• Replace half of the food you eat with fat free goods eg. dressings on salads, cream cheese, diary products, peanut butter etc. and keep on using half of the real thing. You are still cutting back on fat.

• Prepare several meatless meals a week

• Beware of fat substitutes- no in depth or long term studies have been done on the effects of the body

• Do not revamp your whole diet all at one time. Start with one change at a time and when you are comfortable with this, try the next change

• Switch from white rice to brown rice.

• Change from white flour to whole wheat

    The reason that fats are so hard to stay away from is because they have a composition that give food its flavor and fragrance. Long-term energy and a feeling of fullness after a meal are also attributed to fats because they take longer to digest than protein and carbohydrates. ***Unrefined,*** *non-hydrogenated oils are an important source of beneficial fats - they are actually good for you.*

2) Cut Down On Your Sugar Intake - Not All Is Sweet With Sugar

The average North American now consumes about **120 pounds, 17 times as much or approximately 30-33 teaspoons of sugar everyday!** Sugar is hidden in almost every processed food (even to some brands of salt, toothpaste, tea bags and tobacco). [39]

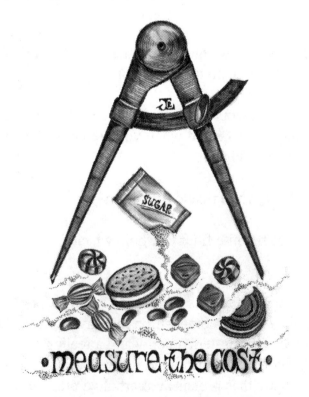

Heart disease, diabetes, and cancer, which were barely evident in the 19th century, seem to have exploded in direct correlation to the increase in sugar usage. Other health conditions related to sugar are yeast, parasitic infections, hypoglycemia, emotional problems, and increased risk of osteoporosis and kidney stones.

Sugar weakens the immune system and evidence now shows that excessive sugar consumption is implicated in more than 60 ailments. Just 100 grams of sugar (in any form) makes white blood cells sluggish within one hour of ingestion. [40]

Excessive sugar interferes with the transport of Vitamin C by blocking absorption or increasing excretion of many minerals.

1)   Sugar reduces the ability of white blood cells to destroy bacteria thereby reducing the body's natural immunity to infection.

2)   Sugar neutralises action of essential fatty acids

3)   Sugar increases the blood glucose level which leads to excess fat production. Excessive fat stores have been linked to colon and breast cancer.

4)   Sugar decreases glucose tolerance which strains the pancreas and potentially leads to hypoglycemia or dia betes mellitus.

5)   Sugar increases blood pressure which could eventually lead to stroke or heart problems.

Tricking Your Taste Buds

If you are trying to cut back on sugar, author/nutritionist Ann Louise Gilleman offers the following tips from *"Get the Sugar Out"* [41]

→   Cut down on salt to lessen cravings for sugar

→   Indulge sweet cravings with fresh fruits or desserts with natural ingredients

→   Treats don't have to be sweet- just new and different

→   Explore taste sensations other than sugary or salty

→   Learn to enjoy food taste as they are

→   Replace candy with nuts, seeds or popcorn as a snack

NOTEWORTHY:

Another good replacement for sugar is **honey**. Honey 1) is high in fructose, which is healthier than the sucrose and glucose found in table sugar. 2) It contains chromium, a mineral required to process sugars. 3) Honey contains bioflavonoids that help the body's self-defence mechanism by fighting infections and also aids in slowing down the aging process. 4) Honey is also a natural antibiotic that when applied on the skin, over cuts, and is beneficial in the prevention of infections.

Beware: *Brown sugar is merely sugar crystals coated with molasses syrup. Just because a product is marked sugarless does not mean that it is low calorie. The biggest misconception about artificial sweeteners is that they have no calories. Sometimes they have as many calories as sugar.*

3) Cut Down On Fast Foods

Have you been super-sizing your fast food meals? It is one of this centuries' best marketing scheme, since everyone wants more for less. In this fast food society it is hard to resist. But, at McDonald's a quarter-pounder with cheese has 530 calories, 30 grams of fat, 13 grams of saturated fat, and 1080 mg. of sodium. Add to this, McDonalds large french fries that have 520 calories, 24 grams of fat, 12 grams of saturated fat and 280 mg. of sodium. [42] Condiments like ketchup and mustard are not included. There is nothing nutritional in this especially for a body that is suffering from CFS and fibromyalgia. Also when you indulge in this food you are not eating the required servings of vegetable and fruits that a person who is chronically ill should be eating. You are also not getting a diet rich in fiber that is so necessary to clean out your colon and remove toxic waste from your body. Your body must have certain nutrients to maintain its fighting strength.

When your immune system is strong, certain designated cells seek out unwanted invaders and promptly get rid of them. When our diet consists mainly of fast foods, we do not give these cells enough fighting ammunition to do the necessary job of defence. These cells become outnumbered, over-whelmed and overburdened and have to defend us on too many fronts. One important thing that you have to remember is, every time you put something into your mouth you must think, "Is this beneficial to my body, can I make this more nutritious, or am I making matters worse for my body to help itself get better? Food is one of the most important aspects of obtaining better health for a CFS person.

4) Increasing Dietary Fiber

In 1996, the USA Federal Drug Administration (FDA) granted manufacturers the right to make specific health claims about Fiber. The proposed health claim states that diets high in fiber may reduce the risk of heart disease. It is the first claim ever permitted to a food by the FDA. Dietary fiber helps to diminish the fat in our blood and decrease blood pressure. Fiber keeps our arteries clean, prevents unwanted weight gain and expedites the elimination of toxins from the intestines.

The liver is constantly trying to clear out the bad cholesterol by dumping it into the intestines. If we ingest enough fiber, our bodies dispose of cholesterol waste rather than reabsorbing it back into the bloodstream. Increasing our fiber intake helps us feel full.

We all know that fiber effects the colon. It passes through the intestines acting as a wet sponge holding and absorbing not only water and toxins but also such compounds as bile acids, which might modify cholesterol metabolism. Fiber, eaten on a regular basis has a buffering effect on gastric acids in the stomach, which suggests some protection of the development of some types of ulcers.

Dietary fiber is the term used for several materials that make up the parts of plants that your body cannot digest. Fiber is classified as soluble or insoluble. Fruits, vegetables, whole-grain foods, beans and legumes are all good sources of dietary fiber.

Insoluble fiber does not appear to help lower blood cholesterol. However, it is an important aid in normal bowel function. Foods high in insoluble fiber include whole-wheat breads, wheat cereals, wheat bran, cabbage, beets, carrots, brussel sprouts, turnips, cauliflower, and apple skin.

BOTTOM LINE:

It is so important that we cleanse our bodies. Fiber helps a CFS patient to rid the body of toxins. Keep thinking in your head "I must eliminate". My cells have been damaged and there is a lot of debris in my body and it absolutely must come out. There are four ways that our body rids the body of toxins:

1)   The lungs
2)   The skin
3)   The kidneys
4)   The intestines

Fiber helps the intestines to cleanse themselves. Remember that almost all CFS patients have intestinal problems. Often times the liver is sluggish which means less production of digestive enzymes. This creates leaky gut syndrome and other digestive disorders. Often times either parasites or clogged intestines will cause a malabsorption syndrome which also is found frequently in chronic fatigue cases. Most CFS patients cannot even absorb the proper nutrients from their food and supplements because their intestines are so malfunctioning. So once again start eating that fiber and make sure that you drink plenty of water (which is what we will elaborate on in the next section).

5) Increase Your Water Intake

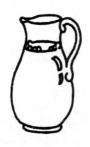

The kidneys cannot function without enough water and when this happens some of their load is dumped onto the liver. One of the liver's primary function is to metabolize stored fat into useable energy for the body. If the liver has to do some of the kidney's work, it cannot function as it was intended. As a result, the liver metabolizes less fat and more fat is stored in the body. The weight loss is stopped.

Constipation

The colon is where all your waste goes. When the body does not receive enough water it takes it from the colon. The result is constipation. When the colon is clean the liver and kidneys can detoxify; the lymph system drains; the lungs can breathe; the skin clears up and the rest of the body feels better.

Fluid Retention

Drinking enough water is the best treatment for fluid retention (edema). When the body receives less water than it needs it holds on to every drop. Water is stored outside the cells and that is why feet, legs and hands swell. Diuretics offer only a temporary solution.

Muscle Tone

By enhancing the muscle's natural ability to contract, water can help the body maintain proper muscle control.

Chose The Cleanest Water

There are different types of water. ***Distilled water*** is tap water that has been boiled until it turns to steam, which is then collected and condensed back into a liquid free of impurities, chemicals and minerals. This process creates flavor-free water. ***Mineral water*** is spring water. It is naturally alkaline, which makes it a natural antacid and a mild diuretic (a substance that increases urination). Bottled water is a better choice than *tap water.*

Drinking water needs to be free from pesticides, pollutants, fertilizers, parasites, and bacteria. ***DRINKING WATER SHOULD BE COLD.*** Studies have shown that cold water is absorbed into the system more quickly and may actually help to burn calories through thermogenesis.

Benefits Of Drinking Water

When the body functions at its optimum, it is getting the water it needs and the fluids are balanced perfectly. There are five modes of action that results:

• The endocrine gland function improves

• Fluid retention is relieved

• More fat is used as fuel because the liver is free to metabolize stored fat

• Natural thirst returns

• There is a loss of hunger overnight

How Much Should We Drink?

A person should drink at least 8 glasses of water a day which is a total of at least 64 ounces a day. An overweight person needs one additional glass for every 25 pounds of excess weight. The amount of water should increase when we exercise or in the summer during hot weather.

Changing Your Supplements

If you have CFS, you need to supplement your diet. As a matter of fact, anyone who is breathing on this planet and not taking antioxidants, vitamins or herbs cannot possibly be getting the protection that one needs in this day and age. But specifically for the CFS patient whose immune system is greatly compromised, supplementation of one's diet is essential. If you think that you can get enough nutrients out of the food that you eat, then you are mistaken. Here are the essential supplements that I recommend for successful treatment of CFS.

Pycnogenol® - The Bark With The Bite

Without the addition of Pycnogenol® to your diet you will not greatly improve from CFS. If you do nothing else, but take Pycnogenol®, your body will respond to the world's #1 antioxidant. In 1993, after my wife suffered for 2 years with CFS, we discovered Pycnogenol®. A friend of mine suggested that Rose-Marie try this pine bark extract from France. Let me tell you

that when you are suffering from CFS you are willing to try anything. All my treatment and advice to my wife was of some help but there was no significant improvement. However, in May 1993 there was a real turn around in Rose-Marie's health after taking Pycnogenol®. I remember her threatening my life if I did not keep supplying her with Pycnogenol®. Pycnogenol® in 1993 was not as readily available as it is today. Friends this is an all-natural product that gives your sick body the kick start that it needs to get better. Other supplements are good but Pycnogenol® is the cream of the crop. Since 1993, my first step in treating CFS is giving Pycnogenol® to my patients. Since that time, I can say with great confidence that Pycnogenol® is the #1 CFS buster!!!

Seven Reasons Why Pycnogenol® Works For CFS Patients

The best known antioxidants in a diet are Vitamin C and E. Additional antioxidants are also found in certain plants, some of which are known as bioflavonoids and minerals. There are thousands of known mixtures of bioflavonoids which enhance the body's ability to absorb Vitamin C. Scientists believe that a diet, rich in these substances can help the body fight and destroy free radicals. Pycnogenol® is one of the most potent bioflavonoids ever discovered. In large part this is due to its outstanding water-solubility and ready absorption into the bloodstream. Pycnogenol® offers these proven benefits to CFS patients:

• Pycnogenol® (pine bark extract) **neutralises** free radicals in the blood stream, and helps **inhibit the formation of free radicals.** Free radicals as we have shown earlier are a major cause of CFS. Pycnogenol literally rust proofs our bodies cells.

• By strengthening the health of the blood vessel walls, circulation is improved in the hands and feet and in the tiny capillaries that feed the eyes, offering strong benefits to smokers, diabetic retinopathy, and varicose veins. Tissues and organs throughout the body that rely on adequate blood flow can be restored to a healthy state and thus reduce edema.

• Pycnogenol® eases allergies by inhibiting the formation of the enzymes that cause allergies. By reducing histamine production, Pycnogenol® helps the arteries resist attack by mutagen which contribute to cardiovascular disease.

• It boosts immunity.

• Pycnogenol® is one of only a few substances that readily crosses the blood - brain barrier to protect the blood vessels in the brain from oxidation. Free radical quenching can take place in the brain. This makes it quite effective for people suffering from CFS to improve general brain function.

• Pycnogenol® actually has the ability to bind to collagen and help collagen fibers rebuild their cross-links to reverse the damage caused by injury and free radical attack. This collagen build-up helps return flexibility and suppleness to skin allowing it to function as an "oral cosmetic". It also has the ability to return flexibility to joint and arteries.

• **There is no question that inflammation plays a key role in the symptoms of Chronic Fatigue Syndrome, the "good news"** for Chronic Fatigue Sufferers is that Pycnogenol® relieves inflammation and also inhibits the processes that lead to inflammation. In addition, Pycnogenol® represses histamine release, which further reduces inflammation.

Saturation Dose

It is important to start taking Pycnogenol® with a saturation dose. 25 mg of Pycnogenol® should be taken for every 25 pounds of body weight. So if you weigh 100 pounds, then you should be taking 100 mg. If you weigh 200 pounds, you should be taking 200mg. This is called a saturation dose.

It is very important that people suffering from CFS take a saturation dose for at least 6 weeks.

Pycnogenol® - The Free Radical Terminator

No matter how many times I review the following list, I become absolutely astounded with what Pycnogenol® can do. We are talking about a natural, totally safe product, that cannot be overused and that substantially improves conditions that were previously thought to be lost causes. This chapter will take you through each one of Pycnogenol's® characteristics along with the disorders that are associated with each point. I will also present you with the testimonials of real people whose suffering was eased as a result of this product. My objective in writing this chapter was not to present you with complicated laboratory studies on Pycnogenol® (although there are many) but, to offer you life stories from real people who have gone through what you may be experiencing right now. I want what you read the following pages and encourage you to take a new direction in your life.

There are nine reasons why Pycnogenol® stands head and shoulders above other antioxidant products on the market to-day:

1)   Pycnogenol® assists in the optimum functioning of all body systems.

2)   Pycnogenol® crosses the blood brain barrier

3)   Pycnogenol® is the most powerful antioxidant known to man. 50 times more powerful than vitamin E, and 20 times more powerful than vitamin C.

4)   Pycnogenol® is bioavailable- your body loves it!

5)   Pycnogenol® is water soluble and completely safe

6)   Pycnogenol® makes vitamin C work better and stay
       longer in our bodies

7)   Pycnogenol® inhibits enzymes such as collagenasc
       and elastase which degrade connective tissue

8)   Pycnogenol® restores blood vessels and fragile
       capillaries

9)   Pycnogenol® does wonders for the skin

Pycnogenol® And Its Effect On The Immune And Respiratory System

   The immune network is a very complex system with
many disorders attributed to it. The diseases range from
diabetes, hypoglycemia, multiple sclerosis, lupus erythe-
matosus, asthma, chronic fatigue syndrome/ fibromyalgia,
yeast infections, viruses, hypothyroidism and allergies. The
immune system is able to recognize and respond to millions of different foreign invaders, referred to as antigens.
An antigen is anything that triggers an immune response.
The chief components of that response are called white
blood cells. There are trillions of white blood cells in the
body at any one time. There are many different classes of
white blood cells. The most notable of these are divided

into three groups, these are T-cells, B-cells, and the macrophages. Abnormalities have been demonstrated in the function of T-cells, B-cells, and macrophages, which indicates some form of disease present. Pycnogenol's® multipurpose action is from its ability to function as a potent antioxidant and also from its role as an extraordinary vitamin C and bioflavonoid helper.

Pycnogenol®, after 20 years of research, has shown to facilitate the immune system by:

1)   acting as an antihistimine

2)   strengthening blood vessels

3)   manufacturing collagen protein - the glue that holds bodily cells together

4)   protecting against bacteria, viruses and infection

5)   assisting in hemoglobin production

6)   stimulating the body's own production of interferon, a powerful anti-viral agent

7)   acting as a diuretic

Pycnogenol® And Viral Infections

Viruses are parasites which depend on nutrients inside the cells of the host for their metabolic and reproductive needs. Viruses are believed to be the cause of the common cold, influenza, smallpox yellow fever, upper respiratory infections, herpes and AIDS. Healthy immune processes are one's best defence. The best way to achieve this is from Pycnogenol® because of its proanthocyanidin-bioflavonoid capabilities. Not only do these compounds protect the cell itself, but, they also help repair the condition of the arteries and capillaries.

Allergies

Allergies occur when the body's immune system overreacts to harmless substances, inhaled or ingested, and are described as a process of inflammation. This process involves free radicals and Pycnogenol® is a free radical scavenger. It is the job of the immune system to be on the alert to recognize, evaluate, neutralize and eliminate invading viruses, bacteria, and other organisms that can cause disease. The immune system can seek these out and then send out histamine as the body's natural defense against invaders to demolish them, before they cause illness. In people with allergies, this immune response goes into "overkill" and does not know when to "shut off" without some kind of external intervention.   At the 1990 Symposium on Pycnogenol®, Dr. D. White of the University of Nottingham reported that Pycnogenol® greatly reduces the formation of histamine by inhibiting the enzyme histidine decarboxylase.

Digestive System

Some of the disorders of this system comprise of ulcerative colitis, spastic colon, stress ulcers, irritable bowel syndrome, and Chrone's disease. Stress ulcers are acute hemorrhagic ulcers of the esophagus, stomach and duodenum that result in serious gastrointestinal bleeding and death. Histamine is involved in the pathogenesis of stress ulcers. Pycnogenol® inhibits the enzyme histamine decarboxylase that is known to lower histamine levels. Pycnogenol® reduces stress ulcers in the stomach and intestine by 82 percent because it prevents excessive histamine release. In 1990, researchers in Great Britain confirmed this and reported on the Pycnogenol® anti-stress action and how it prevents ulcer formation.

Premenstrual Syndrome (PMS)

PMS is one of the most common problems affecting women during their reproductive years. PMS rarely corrects itself on its own. Approximately 50% of menstruating women suffer from cyclical bouts of fluid retention, painful swollen breasts, inflated stomach, puffy face, undefined pelvic pain, weight gain, functional disturbances in the legs, irritation, depression and headaches. These symptoms occur from an increased sensitivity to normal physiological variations in estrogen and progesterone levels. Women suffering from PMS were given 200mg. of Pycnogenol® a day. In 61 percent of the women, the physical disorders disappeared after two cycles. In 79 percent of the women, the physical disorders disappeared after four cycles.

The Blood Brain Barrier

I always have a little chuckle when I see wide-eyed expressions on some of my patients faces when I state that Pycnogenol® crosses the blood-brain barricr. This particular medical assertion has such a dramatic, life-altering tone to it that I can be assured of their complete and undivided attention for the rest of my explanation. Rest assured, there is nothing that complicated about it. The blood-brain barrier is in place to protect the brain's fragile capillaries, brain matter and nerve endings. Like a bouncer kicking out under-agers in a bar, the barrier does not allow just any nutrient to go through. Most of us take drugs that cross the blood-brain barrier on a regular basis such as cold and allergy medications. These drugs usually have some side effects such as drowsiness and lethargy. If, on the package, the written instructions indicate that you shouldn't drive a motorized vehicle, you are taking a drug that crosses that barrier. Pycnogenol® is powerful enough to cross the blood-brain barrier and of particular significance is the fact that there are absolutely no side effects. Keep in mind that most natural products are not strong enough to cross that barrier. The fact that Pycnogenol® is able to do so means that it is effective for use against Attention Deficit Disorder, Alzeihemer's and Chronic Fatigue Syndrome. The following information on each of these disorders will give you a better idea about Pycnogenol's® ability to cross the blood-brain barrier.

Powerful Antioxidant

As I have devoted a section in this book to free radical damage, I will not go into great detail here. Suffice it to say that Pycnogenol® is the most powerful antioxidant ever discovered. What this means in terms of our health is that Pycnogenol® is the best rust proofing, anti-aging nutrient for our cells that money can buy.

Bioavailability

Although a lengthy word, its meaning is quite simple: it means that Pycnogenol® is easily absorbed in your blood stream. Did you know that most nutrients have very poor bioavailability? Vitamin C, for instance, is excreted from your body within 4-6 hours after ingestion. Pycnogenol®, on the other hand, stays in your body for up to 72 hours and is therefore able to go to work big time on the cell. In fact, if you decided to take a saliva test just 20 minutes after taking Pycnogenol®, the result would indicate that it would already be working in your blood stream.

Water Solubility

Pycnogenol® is water soluble and completely safe. In other words, what your body doesn't need, it excretes. Fat soluble nutrients like vitamin E can be toxic if too much is taken. A participant in a recent study on Pycnogenol® took 80 tablets in a day and the result was that he experienced no side effects. Pycnogenol® has years of scientific research to back up this claim of safety.

A Potentiator Of Vitamin C

One of Pycnogenonol's® most remarkable feats is its ability to improve upon the efficacy of vitamin C. Pycnogenol's® synergistic association with vitamin C causes the vitamin to remain in the body longer, enabling it to travel to cell and collagen levels. What I suggest to my patients is that if they feel a cold coming on, to double their dose of Pycnogenol® and take a little more vitamin C. Many patients have told me that since they started on Pycnogenol® they no longer get colds. An even more effective way of staving off colds is to take Pycnogenol® with Acerola, the purest and strongest form of vitamin C in the world. Many patients who used to get 2-3 nasty colds a year, now after taking Pycnogenol® may only get one mild sniffle a year. Try and double your daily dose of Pycnogenol® for a few days, at the first sign of a cold.

Inhibitor Of Enzymes Collagenes Collagenes An Elastase

Enzymes like collagenese and elastase degrade connective tissue in the body which effects areas like the joints and skin. As anyone suffering from arthritic problems can attest, it has been a problem where treatments have not been forthcoming. Yet, it was discovered that Pycnogenol®

works as a natural anti-inflammatory and also helps to re-build joints. Best of all, it decreases the enzymes that cause pain to joints. The results have been very encouraging for people with rheumatoid arthritis and chronic osteo- arthritis. In addition, I encourage athletes to use Pycnogenol® to prevent and restore joint damage.

Restores Blood Vessels And Fragile Capillaries

Its ability to restore blood vessels and fragile capillaries in organs and tissue all throughout our bodies makes it indispensable to our health. Pycnogenol® is so effective in inhibiting inflammation because it increases blood circulation. In addition, it helps in removing inflammation which causes varicose veins and tired leg syndrome. Tired leg syndrome, by the way, is often related to sleep disorders. Pycnogenol® helps to rebuild the collagen level of the inner lining of your arteries and capillaries. Free radicals therefore have far less chance of hitting those vessels and damaging them because of their new strength and more resiliencies. Cholesterol in itself, does not cause problems until it starts sticking to blood vessels, eventually causing clogging of the arteries and cardiovascular disease. While the case histories of patients who have had their cholesterol lowered after taking Pycnogenol® are numerous, I will introduce you to the most dramatic case that I have ever encountered.

A patient of mine started taking Pycnogenol® after he was told by his cardiologist that he needed bypass surgery because of four blocked arteries, one of which had a 99 per cent block. At this point, his doctor was willing to try anything and encouraged my patients's use of Pycnogenol®. A couple of months after taking Pycnogenol® he went back to his cardiologist and what the doctor witnessed almost knocked him over the clogging of his patient's arteries had decreased somewhere between 60 to 80 per cent. The doctor also noticed that this man's stress tests were within normal limits and that his energy level had improved to such an extent that he was able to play hockey again. All of this from a man who was so sick that he had to take one full year off from work.

CHAPTER FOURTEEN

Seeing Is Believing

We have recently completed a ten case study on CFS, free radical damage and Pycnogenol®. One of our findings, that CFS was a free radical disorder, was consistent with that of Dr. Ally, author of "The Canary and Chronic Fatigue Syndrome". We found that after CFS participants had taken the saturation dose of Pycnogenol® for the six-week period, there was a 60 per cent overall improvement in the most debilitating of all symptoms - fatigue. We also learned that brain functions and cognitive abilities in CFS patients were improved by 70 per cent, short term memory and attention span had been heightened by 60 per cent and as the brain was restored to its near normal state. Sleeping patterns and sleep disturbances improved by 70 per cent. In actuality, there was some kind of noted improvement in every one of the people that voluntarily took part in our study. The skepticism of those who had tried every kind of natural product known to man was forgotten as participants began to feel better. Therefore, the summary of our clinical findings after six weeks suggest a marked diminishment of fatigue primarily due to Pycnogenol's® powerful antioxidant properties and its ability to cross the blood-brain barrier, thereby protecting brain cells. The blood-brain barrier is the body's natural defence against some compounds that normally circulate in the blood to which brain cells are sensitive. These compounds may not damage other cells in the body or even be needed by the other cells, but the brain filters out as many unnecessary compounds as it can. Pycnogenol® is a natural non-drug product and by its very properties brings oxygen with it through the blood-brain barrier, thus improving mental alertness. The following is a summary of each one of the ten participants in our CFS study. Each patient seemed to have one or more major complaint besides fatigue.

PARTICIPANT #1

This woman with CFS also suffered from an allergic condition called hypersensitive pneumonitis as well as relentless environmental sensitivities. Her condition improved 50 per cent after she completed six weeks on a saturation dose of Pycnogenol®. The immune system is made up of cells with the capacity for recognizing, evaluating, neutralizing and eliminating alien material. Allergies are described as a process of inflammation known to be a disorder of the immune system. In an allergic response, our immune system spots an antigen and sends out histamine as the body's natural defence against invaders. While the immune system has no problems releasing histamine, it does not recognize any signal to turn it off. The histamine proceeds on overkill and does not cease without some kind of external intervention. This process involves free radicals and Pycnogenol® is a free radical scavenger. At the 1990 International Symposium on Pycnogenol®, Doctor D. White, at the University of Nottingham, reported that Pycnogenol® greatly reduces this free radical process - the formation of histamine.

PARTICIPANT #2 AND #3

Both diagnosed with CFS, participants 2 and 3 experienced severe migrating joint pain and muscle weakness and fibromyalgia.Today, there are some 50-60 diseases associated with free radical damage and fibromyalgia has recently been added to the list. Free radicals are highly reactive unstable molecules with unattached electrons. The chemical nature of these molecules result in their immediate reaction with one of the body's normal chemicals and have been shown to initiate damage to the joint membrane. This destruction causes chain reactions releasing thousands of free radicals, which in turn, causes inflammation. Pycnogenol® helps reduce the inflammation, which is the primary cause behind the painful symptoms associated with CFS by quenching some of the free radicals involved at the sight of inflammation. The second participant's pain and muscle weakness had abated by 100 per cent after the six-week period on Pycnogenol®.

PARTICIPANT #4

Participant 4, a CFS patient, suffered from tachycardia (irregular heartbeat) and elevated blood pressure. The results of a new John Hopkins study shows that CFS is strongly linked to a common and potentially treatable abnormality of blood pressure regulation. This does not negate the fact that the adrenal glands have been affected, the culprit being free radical damage. After six weeks on Pycnogenol® her tachycardia and blood pressure symptoms had receded by 80 per cent. According to Dr. Ruwe, Pycnogenol® has an anti hypertensive affect by inhibiting the angiotensin which is a converting enzyme. This exhibits an inhibitory effect on adrenaline induced platelet aggregation. In addition, we believe that this contributes to protection against hypertension.

PARTICIPANT #5- DIABETIC RETINOPATHY

Participant 5 suffered from Chronic Fatigue Syndrome and had severe childhood diabetes. Before her participation in my study, she had experienced severe hemorrhaging behind the eyes, which required laser surgery. Since taking Pycnogenol®, there has been a dramatic improvement in her eye condition and she has even been encouraged by her optomologist to continue taking Pycnogenol®. Since Pycnogenol® reduces vascular fragility, its protective influence extends to the fragile capillaries of the eyes, a shielding effect that is pronounced for more than eight hours. Pycnogenol® produces a more prolonged recovery in capillary resistance compared to most bioflavonoids. Dr.Sibbel, at the Second International Pycnogenol® Symposium, has shown that this is probably due to Pycnogenol's® sheltering effect on vitamin C and its adherence to collagen. For the past several years, Pycnogenol® has been licensed in France for treating Diabetic Retinopathy after clinical studies established that it was a viable treatment. Dr. G. Manard and his colleagues conducted a study of 40 patients. The patients were given 80-120 mg of Pycnogenol® for a week followed by 40-80 mg daily for 1-4 months. The microbleeding of the capillaries decreased remarkably in 90 per cent of the patients and their eye-sight improved noticeably. Furthermore, Professor Saracco of the Clinic of Ophthalmology in Marseilles studied 60 patients and confirmed that Pycnogenol not only improved Diabetic Retinopathy and Hypertensive Retinopathy, it also diminished loosening of the Retina. German medical professor and director of the university eye clinic in Wurzburg, Dr. HCW Leydhecker found that Pycnogenol® compares favourably with all other current treatments for Diabetic Retinopathy. Dr. Leydhecker compared the effectiveness of Pycnogenol® and the drug Dexium, which is used routinely to suppress the progress of Diabetic Retinopathy. There were 16 patients in each group (a placebo group was not included because the patients were referred to the study from a private practice). Seven university professors evaluated the photographs of the patients' Retinas before and after treatment without being aware of which patients were taking Pycnogenol®. After 6 months of treatment, both compounds were found to be equally effective.

PARTICIPANT #6

Before entering into the study, Participant 6 had been referred to a neurologist who had the patient undergo an EEG (a device used to record and measure electrical wave activity of the brain). She had been suffering from Petite Mal seizures which can be a rare symptom of Chronic Fatigue Syndrome. Pycnogenol's® ability to transport oxygen across the blood-brain barrier throughout the brain, stimulates blood circulation as well as strengthen and restore flexibility to arterial walls. Perhaps this is what terminated her Petite Mal occurrences. Since that time, she has continued to take Pycnogenol® and has had no further seizures.

PARTICIPANT #7

Participant 7 is a young woman who suffered from CFS. After she had completed her six week saturation interval, she had a remarkable resurgence of energy, consisting of an overall degree of well-being and a heightened degree of unconfused cognitive functioning. Up until recently, we knew that blood flow in the brain was disrupted but we did not know to what extent. The continuity of blood flow in the brain of CFS patients can now be measured by using a" Spect" scanner. This new technology involves the use of one of two radioactive substances that cross the blood-brain barrier, permeating the spaces of the brain — one that is inhaled or one that is injected. Dr. Ishmahel Mena, Professor of Radiology at the University of California, studied 46, CFS patients using Spect scans. All of these patients were found to have diminished blood flow in four areas of the brain including the area that influences thinking and learning. When there is not enough blood flowing through the brain, there is insufficient oxygen for the brain to function properly.

Pycnogenol® has also been scientifically proven to enhance the efficacy of vitamin C. I believe this young woman benefited from Pycnogenol's® biovailability which helps cells absorb, utilize and prolong the effectiveness of vitamin C. Furthermore, Pycnogenol® is 20 times more powerful than vitamin C as an antioxidant. It is the protective effect of vitamin C that results in more of it being available to enter cells. Antioxidants combine readily with oxygen and neutralize oxygen radicals, thus becoming free radical terminators. This initiates a chain reaction resulting in strengthened capillaries, improved blood circulation in the brain resulting in a higher level of energy and cognitive capabilities.

PARTICIPANT #8

Participant 8 suffered from unbearable attacks of panic. Her symptoms included sudden dizziness and profuse sweating as well as the tightening of chest and stomach muscles — all in response to what others would consider only little things, like driving her car through a busy intersection or riding up an elevator. After the participant had taken the required saturation dose of Pycnogenol® for six weeks, she discovered that her panic attacks had disappeared. Pycnogenol's® superantioxidant and bioflavonoid qualities helped it to adhere to the collagen fibres in the blood vessels thus restoring resilience and flexibility to them. The revitalized collagen and elasticity helped renew the impermeability of blood vessel walls which succeeding in eliminating capillary leaking. The rejuvenated blood vessel system thus improves circulation to the brain. The participant has continued to take Pycnogenol® and has not had a single panic attack since.

PARTICIPANT #9

Participant 9 is a 50 year old, with a type A personality who was diagnosed with CFS. While her forced decelerated lifestyle left her feeling very frustrated, she had no choice but to adjust just as a prisoner conforms to his jail cell. Although she rested, and slept a full 2/3 of her day, she felt as exhausted when she woke up in the morning, as when she went to bed at night. The additional stress of fibrocystis did not help the situation. For the six-week period, she took the saturation dose of Pycnogenol® and her inability to fall asleep diminished. She stopped waking up 2-3 times a night disorientated and ceased tossing and turning in bed. One of the ways researchers' measure CFS patients' brain wave, is to monitor electrical activity generated by the brain. A researcher in Charlotte, North Carolina, Myra Preston, states that brain wave patterns seen in CFS patients are exactly opposite of the brain wave patterns of healthy people. When a healthy person is awake and functioning the brain produces primarily a combination of alpha and beta waves. CFS patients appear to be stuck in theta waves - their brain produce high levels of the brain wave associated with drowsiness, even when they are awake. The result is that CFS patients are never fully awake and able to function intellectually; neither can they fall deeply asleep. Pycnogenol's® ability to cross the blood brain barrier and resulting improved blood and oxygen supply probably provide the answer to Pycnogenol's® success in participant # 9 symptoms.

PARTICIPANT #10

This young woman agonized over recurring yeast infections which is often a symptom of CFS. Presence of yeast can stress the immune system and over a period of time can cause it to become so overworked that it becomes unable to resist the entry of unwanted invaders. Yet, contrary to popular belief, an anti-fungal therapy is not always the answer. The cream partially disintegrates the cell wall of a yeast organism, rupturing the yeast cell, allowing its inner contents to escape and pass through the absorptive membrane of the intestinal wall, causing low-level immune challenge and detoxification crisis. Pycnogenol® helps to increase capillary function thus improving the flow of oxygen. Since oxygen is an important detoxifyer, waste organisms are destroyed.

(43) (44) (45) (46) (47) (48)

Recommended Supplements For CFS

Coenzyme Q 10

People who suffer with Chronic Fatigue Syndrome have vitamin and nutritional deficiencies. Coenzyme Q10 is a naturally occurring substance that is fat soluble with characteristics that are common to vitamins. Coenzyme Q10 is one of the substances in the chain of reactions, which produces energy in the metabolism of food. Almost every cell of a living organism contains CoQ10 because of its necessity for energy production. CoQ10 helps drive the mitochondrial energy production vital to all body functions and is a strong antioxidant which protects LDL -low density protein- (the good cholesterol) against oxidation. Coenzyme Q10 stimulates the immune system and helps lower blood pressure. The functioning of all organs depends on each cell having adequate levels of CoQ10 to provide life-sustaining energy. The gastrointestinal tract best absorbs it when taken with meals. The usual dosage for a person who suffers from CFS is anywhere from 60-200mg./day.

Evening Primrose Oil

The Evening Primrose Oils' most active ingredient is Gamma Linolenic Acid (GLA) which is an essential fatty acid (EFA). Our bodies do not produce EFA's and therefore must be obtained from our diet (cold water fish such as cod, trout, salmon, shark) and from nutritional supplements. These fish contain high quantities of omega-3 fatty acids which can act as an anti-inflammatory and even diminish allergic responses. Dr. Michael D.Wintter and Dr. Peter Behan has shown some encouraging results using Evening Primrose Oil on Chronic Fatigue patients. The controlled study for EFA's was conducted at the Glasglow Southern General Hospital in which 68 patients were given 8 capsules a day for a total of three months. A control group was given a placebo and their overall condition relative to that when beginning the trial was assessed after three months. Out of the 68 patients taking Evening Primrose Oil, 53 felt they had improved and 31 out of the 68 felt they had "much improved". Dr. Les Simpson of New Zealand a leading CFS researcher recommends no less than 8 capsules a day of Evening Primrose Oil.

Vitamin C

Vitamin C maintains immunity and can prevent many types of viral and bacterial infections. This water-soluble vitamin cannot be made by the human body, so our main source is from food. The best benefit of taking vitamin C comes when it is taken along with Pycnogenol® since Pycnogenol® helps vitamin C to work more efficiently in the body. Pycnogenol® can also regenerate used vitamin C into active vitamin C. Vitamin C, in turn can recycle used vitamin E into active vitamin E. When the immune system is in such a low state of functioning that antioxidants such as Pycnogenol and Vitamin C are at the top of the list of "must take" supplements.

Bovine Colostrum

The #1 killer in the world today is immune disease. Immune deficiencies, auto-immune diseases, heart disease, cancer, allergies, infections, diabetes, ulcers, even aging is immune related. Colostrum is the first milk from the mammary glands of a mother, in a time frame from 24-48 hours after birth. It is mother-nature's perfect combination of growth factors that fight disease and infection by protecting the body from certain viruses, bacteria, allergens and toxins. In humans it transmits disease immunity and stimulates normal healthy growth. This colostrum is from a cow, which is accepted by all other mammals, including man. It is also another step in the return to health and a better quality of life for those suffering from CFS.

Oil Of Oregano

This is a relatively new discovery. Oil of Oregano is the essential oil of the wild oregano plant, which is produced by steam distillation. The oil is extracted from the crushed dry leaves and flowers of various species of oregano, which grow wild on the hillsides, mountains, and in the forests of various regions throughout the world. This is the true oregano - not the spice that you find in your grocery store. This "wild oregano" is rich in essential oils. Oil of Oregano has been tested by researchers and has been found to have:

• Significant antifungal and antibacterial activity.

• Possesses significant antiviral powers

• Parasites fall victim to the intense power of oil of oregano

• Exerts powerful anti-inflammatory actions

• Oil of Oregano is a natural anesthetic and is invaluable in the treatment of various painful lesions and pain disorders

• Oil of oregano can destroy all varieties of fungi and yeasts whether they are on the skin or within the body. Millions of people, especially those who suffer from Chronic Fatigue Syndrome are afflicted with fungal infections, internal and external. A fungus is a type of microbe that lives off of dead or dying tissue. This is why fungi commonly affect the skin. The skin is constantly shedding layers of dead cells. Antibiotics are the major factor in the cause of fungal infestation and are certainly the leading cause of acute fungal infections of the vagina, intestines and mouth. Fungi can also be directly due to the type of diet that the North American eats. Fungi feed primarily upon one substance: sugar. Alcohol is another stimulant for fungal growth. Birth control pills also help to multiply fungal growth. Fungi brings about immune suppression. This is done by the toxins that they give off to poison our immune system. They can also change their cellular wall structure to evade destruction by the white blood cells. This is the way that they continue to grow and advance into new territory. The primary purpose of fungi is to disable the immune system to maintain their preservation.

Changing Your Exercise Philosophy

Increase Your Exercising

I can almost see your face now. Some of you are saying. "Hey doc I can't even get out of bed, so how do you expect me to exercise?" Well here's how. I don't want you to exercise until you have started this regeneration program for at least 21 days. Keep in mind, that I am not going to ask you to run a marathon or beat Arnold Schwarzenegger in arm wrestling. Keeping with our philosophy to eliminate and regenerate, exercise will now play an important part.

Exercise Philosophy

The lifestyle of people on the North American continent has been determined to be major contributing factors in diseases such as diabetes, hypoglycemia, heart disease, and cancer. The most commonly cited factors are inadequate fiber intake, excessive consumption of fats, ingestion of refined sugar and the lack of exercise.

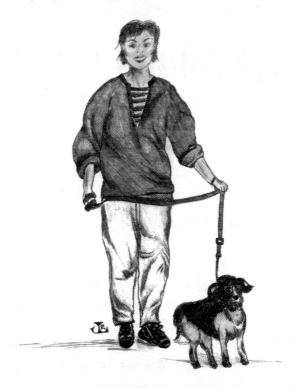

There are many beneficial health reasons for exercising:

→   Aids in fending off health problems such as heart difficulties, diabetes and improve quality of life for those suffering from Chronic Fatigue Syndrome

→   Exercise helps promote sleep. Any help in sleeping for CFS suffers patient is great.

→   Coping with stress is made easier when exercising

→   Exercise is a great plus for your mental health and improving self-esteem - something that is so needed when struggling with CFS

→   Assists the body in slowing down the aging process (how to age gracefully)

→   Exercising is most beneficial for muscle strength and joint flexibility

→   Physical activity is a natural immune system booster and can give the edge needed when the body is fighting off an infection.

Take It Easy

The idea of exercise in CFS is to start slowly. Every day, after 21 days of commencing our lifestyle changes, try and do at least 5-10 minutes of either walking, biking or swimming. You must not jog. Running will deplete your system too quickly and will actually do more harm than good. After another two or three weeks, try and increase your exercise program to 20 minutes. Other good forms of healthy exercise for CFS patients are stretching and a form of pool exercise called aqua-fit which is low impact and easy on the muscles and joints.

Rose-Marie's Story (My Wife)

I am presently a mother of four children, grandmother of three, and a Registered Nurse. I had always stated that if I ever found anything that helps make me feel like a human being again, even if it means swallowing a snake whole, because someone said it would help, I"ll shout it from the rooftop; "Well here is my roof top!"

I did, at on time, start out as a perfectly normal, seemingly healthy human being, but somewhere around the summer of 1991, all that changed. Like everyone else who has been diagnosed with Chronic Fatigue Syndrome, I can remember the exact moment when the general feeling of well-being started to become a distant memory. This was replaced by the awareness of a constant weight of unnatural tiredness, which seemed to wash over me through the day, along with migrating muscle and joint pain.

Initial Onset Of Illness

I led a very active life and was physically fit, running three miles every day and five miles on the weekend. In the summer of 1991, I was diagnosed with allergies never before experienced. By October I was hospitalized with hypersensitive pneumonitis and severe asthma. We eventually sold our house because I could not maintain the multi-levels or even do the stairs, so we sold the "dream" home that we had built and moved into a condominium.

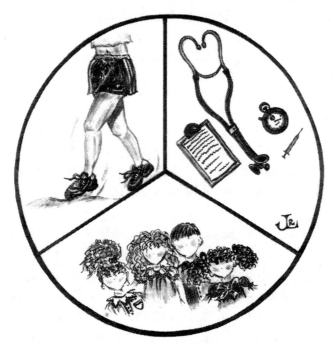

Puzzling Symptoms

Other features were starting to manifest themselves at this time, besides the bone weary tiredness. And muscle aches and joint pain. The mind felt like it has a thick heavy blanket spread over it and mental processes were very slow with short-term memory loss. Severe eye pain became a daily part of life. Gastro-intestinal problems started to occur. Severe distress when digesting food, bloatedness, alternating between diarrhea and constipation led my doctor to start me on medication for the stomach. Anti-inflammatory for the painful muscles and sulfa drugs for the constant bladder and kidney infections were prescribed.

I was also on Prednisone to keep the immune system from going into overkill because of the allergies. Always being an active person, I suddenly had to run a household, and raise four children from the bed and couch. After one year of being on a medical merry-go-round, A diagnosis was confirmed, but frustration set in at an all time high. They were now able to diagnosis Chronic Fatigue Syndrome but they did no have any formal treatment program.

Pycnogenol® - Answer To Prayer

I will never forget the day, a Thursday, in May 1993, that drastically changed the course of my life, at that time. I think of it as a miracle, direct from heaven. A friend of my husband's, a chiropractor, sent me two bottles of an antioxidant with a name I couldn't even pronounce – Pycnogenol". I was so desperate, that I read the note he sent on how to take it – one tablet for every 25 pounds – and downed it without even reading the information or knowing what it was. Friday and Saturday I continued with the same dosage. It wasn't until early Sunday morning, when I awoke, that I noticed a change. I did not feel my usual, deathly ill self. This was when I went and read the information that was sent to me on this pine bark extract. Over the following weeks the transformation was remarkable. The thick heavy blanket over my brain started to lift for the first time in years. To have a clear, consistent thought was simply delightful. The muscle aches and joint pain diminished daily. Momentary forgetfulness subsided. Several months after starting on Pycnogenol" my level of daily living had risen a number of degrees. I still go through the occasional flare-ups, but they are not frequent, do not last so long, and they do not incapacitate me.

I am living proof that my husband's six week program really works. It is very important as a CFS and Fibromyalgia sufferer that you take charge of your body.

The Vicious Circle

Written By My Daughter Stacey Lawrence

Morning's here - Did I even sleep? I can hardly lift my head!

I'll force myself up anyway - with eyes that are puffy red.

Is it Monday, Tuesday or even Wednesday? I can't seem to recall.

For small details and peoples names are the blurriest of all!

Think I used to start my day with one long three mile run

Now I live with muscle pain and I've only just begun

Not only do I feel so weak - but I have pain in every joint

Why live on aspirin everyday? I figure what's the point?

So what's the problem anyway- is what my doctor said

These symptoms you are experiencing- they must be in your head

All my hopes of one day feeling completely like myself

Lie solely on my research to restore me back to health

Now in hopes to make my long story short

I tried all kinds of natural products - one of every sort

So listen when i tell you, and now it is your call

For me the return to good health became Pycnogenol®

Summary of Course of Action

In this book my husband and I want to let you know the steps that I have taken to a better quality of life and much improved health:

1) If you have been tired for several months without any real energy and suffering from other bizarre symptoms, you should suspect the start of CFS.

2) Gather all the information you can on this disorder because **half of the battle is understanding what you are suffering from.**

3) Start on the saturation dose of Pycnogenol®. Some people after the initial dose can cut back to two or three tablets a day. Most CFS sufferers remain on their saturation dose indefinitely.

4) Start on the supplements listed in chapter 15. It is by taking them consistently over a period of time that your immune system will be built back up. Rome wasn't built in a day, neither can your immune system be rebooted in a day. It is a slow, gradual process.

5) Concentrate on cleaning up your diet. You are not what you eat, but what you can absorb. If nutrients

cannot get through to your cells because of poor digestion then neither can your supplements bring nutrition and energy to your cells that desperately need them. A parasite or colonic cleanse will be of the utmost benefit. **Digest Enzymes and Lactobacillus Acidophilus** with each meal will help with breaking down the food and will assist the body in utilizing the nutrients better.

6)   Increase your water intake gradually and work up to 2 litres a day.

7)   Increase your fiber intake and work up to 40 grams a day.

8)   Clear up the yeast infection with oil of oregano and cutting drastically back on sugar intake.

9)   Exercise is of extreme importance. Start at 5 minutes a day and as you increase toleration and muscle strength work up to 30 minutes a day.

10)   Control your sleep disorder instead of it controlling you. Take Dr. Martin Kava Calm which includes Valerian Root and Passion Flower, all natural with no day after side effects. Melatonin is also another great sleep inducer.

11)   Do muscle stretching exercises for the fibromyalgia pain, twice a day. The best time is in the morning when the stiffness is at its worst and at night just

before bedtime since there is nothing like night time fibromyalgia pain to waken you up and keep you awake for the rest of the night. The best place to ob tain these stretches is from a chiropractor. I know that these stretching exercises given to me by my son (a chiropractor) really helped me.

12) Have a live blood cell analysis done (if possible) and then another one 6 months later as comparison to check on improvement.

13) Allergies will come under control if the supplements are consistently taken along with pyc pyc and more pyc (pycnogenol® which is what singularly helped me). The allergy food elimination test also is a great deal of help. If there is a food that you suspect that your are allergic to, eliminate it from your diet for three weeks. After three weeks eat some of this food and see how you feel. Most times it is some of the most common foods that we eat every day that we are allergic to. If you are having a hard time staying away from the food that you have decided to elimi nate, then this is also a good indication that you have an allergy to this food.

Synopsis of What Happens in A Typical CFS Patient

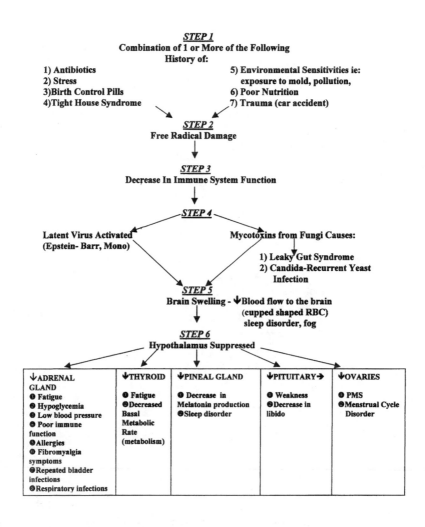

STEP 1
Combination of 1 or More of the Following
History of:

1) Antibiotics
2) Stress
3) Birth Control Pills
4) Tight House Syndrome

5) Environmental Sensitivities ie:
   exposure to mold, pollution,
6) Poor Nutrition
7) Trauma (car accident)

STEP 2
Free Radical Damage

STEP 3
Decrease In Immune System Function

STEP 4

Latent Virus Activated
(Epstein- Barr, Mono)

Mycotoxins from Fungi Causes:

1) Leaky Gut Syndrome
2) Candida-Recurrent Yeast
   Infection

STEP 5
Brain Swelling - ↓Blood flow to the brain
(cupped shaped RBC)
sleep disorder, fog

STEP 6
Hypothalamus Suppressed

↓ADRENAL GLAND	↓THYROID	↓PINEAL GLAND	↓PITUITARY→	↓OVARIES
❶ Fatigue	❶ Fatigue	❶ Decrease in Melatonin production	❶ Weakness	❶ PMS
❷ Hypoglycemia	❷ Decreased Basal Metabolic Rate (metabolism)	❷ Sleep disorder	❷ Decrease in libido	❷ Menstrual Cycle Disorder
❸ Low blood pressure				
❹ Poor immune function				
❺ Allergies				
❻ Fibromyalgia symptoms				
❼ Repeated bladder infections				
❽ Respiratory infections				

References

(1)   Healthwatch, R&T Press, Volume 1, Issue 4, Page 2

(2)   A.W. Martin, Chronic Fatigue Syndromeronic, Free Radical Damage
       and Pycnogenol®, Lasalle University, Mandeville, Louisanna; 1996.

(3)   Rosenbaum, M. and M. Susser, Solving The Puzzle of Chronic
       Fatigue Syndrome, Life Services Press, Tacoma, WA, 1992.

(4)   Hart, A; The Hidden Link Between Adrenalin and Stress, Word
       Publishing, Dallas, Texas, 1991, Pages 3-15.

(5)   Hart, A; The Hidden Link Between Adrenalin and Stress, Word
       Publishing, Dallas, Texas, 1991, Pages 3-15.

(6)   Todd, G. Nutritional, Health and Disease, Schiffer Publishing,
       Atglen Penn, 1985, Pages 50-55

(7)   Toronto Star, August, 1998, Section D, Page 85

(8)   Goldstein, J. "How Do I Diagnosis A Patient With Chronic Fatigue
       Syndrome?" The Clinical and Scientific Basis of Myalgic
       Encephalomyelitis, Chronic Fatigue Syndrome, Nightingale Research
       Foundation, Ottawa, 1992

(9)   Schmidt, M; Tired of Being Tired, Overcoming Chronic Fatigue
       Syndrome and Low Energy, Frog Ltd, Berkley, CA., 1995

(10)   Ostrum, N., 50 Things You Should Know About The Chronic Fatigue
       Syndrome Epidemic, St. Martin's Paperbacks, New York, N.Y., 1993.

(11)   Rosenbaum, M&M. Susser, Solving The Puzzle of Chronic Fatigue
       Syndrome, Life Services Press, Tacoma, WA, page 37, 1996.

(12)   Costantini, A.V. MD., Wieland, H. MD & Qvick, L. MD, Prevention of
       Breast Cancer -Hope at Last, Verlag Publishing, Freiburg,Germany,1998.

(13)   Ostrum, N., 50 Things You Should Know About The Chronic Fatigue
       Syndrome Epidemic, St. Martin's Paperbacks, New York, N.Y., 1993.

(14)   Simpson, L, "The Role of Nondescocytic Erthrocytes in the Pathogenis of Myalgia Encephalomyelitis/CFS", The Clinical and Scientific Basis of Myalgia Encephalomyelites/CFS, Nightingale Foundation, Ottawa, Canada, 1992

(15)   Ostrum, N., 50 Things You Should Know About The Chronic Fatigue Syndrome Epidemic, St. Martin's Paperbacks, New York, N.Y., 1993.

(16)   Rosenbaum, M&M. Susser, Solving The Puzzle of Chronic Fatigue Syndrome, Life Services Press, Tacoma, WA, page 37, 1996.

(17)   Rosenbaum, M&M. Susser, Solving The Puzzle of Chronic Fatigue Syndrome, Life Services Press, Tacoma, WA, page 37, 1996.

(18)   Todd, G. Nutritional, Health and Disease, Schiffer Publishing, Atglen Penn, 1985, Pages 50-55

(19)   Cooper, K, The Antioxidant Revolution, Thomas Nelson, Nashville, Ten, 1994.

(20)   Arstilla, A, "Pycnogenol®-A Free Radical Terminator (FRT) in Humans", The 2nd International Pycnogenol® Symposium, M.W. International Inc., Biarritz, France, 1995.

(21)   Ali, M., The Canary and Chronic Fatiguetigue, Lifespan Press, Denville, N.J., 1995

(22)   Barczak,C., "Live Blood Analysis", Health Naturally Magazine, August/September 1996, 27.

(23)   A.W. Martin, Chronic Fatigue Syndrome, Free Radical Damage and Pycnogenol®, Lasalle University, Mandeville, Louisanna; 1996.

(24)   Cooper, K, The Antioxidant Revolution, Thomas Nelson, Nashville, Ten, 1994

(25)   Todd, G. Nutritional, Health and Disease, Schiffer Publishing, Atglen, Penn, 1985

(26)   A.W. Martin, Chronic Fatigue Syndrome, Free Radical Damage and Pycnogenol®, Lasalle University, Mandeville, Louisanna; 1996.

(27)   Hart, A., The Hidden Link Between Adrenalin and Stress, Word Publishing, Dallas, Texas, 1991, pages 3-15

(28)   Teitelbaum, Dr. Jacob, MD., "From Fatigued to Fantastic", Avery Publishing Group, 1996.

(29)   Babal, K., "Chronic Fatiguetigue Syndromeronic Fatigue Syndrome-The Nutritional Approach", Health and Healing, Fall, 1995: 6-7

(30)   Donsbach, K, Hypogylycemia and Diabetes, Rockland Corp, Santa Monica,CA., 1993

(31)   Miller, B, Understanding Chronic Fatigue Syndrome, BMC, Dallas, Texas, 1991

(32)   Schmidt, R, " Tired of Being Tired, Overcoming Chronic Fatigue and Low Energy, Frog Ltd, Berkley, CA, 1995.

(33)   Donsback, D, Alsleben, M, Sysyemic Candidiasis and CFS, Don et als, Santa Monica, CA, 1992

(34)   Culbert, M. CFS Conquering the Crippler, C and C Communications, San Diego, CA, 1993

(35)   Rosenbaum, M. Susser, Solving The Puzzle of Chronic Fatigue Syndrome, Life Services Press, Tacoma, Wa, 1992

(36)   Pederson, G., Wilson, M., Seeds of Life, Charwood Publishing, Texas, 1997.

(37)   Rona Z., "Overlooked Causes of Chronic Fatigue", Health Naturally, Feb/March, 1996, pages 7-9

(38)   Goldberg, B, Chronic Fatigue, Fibromyalgia and Environmental Illness, Future Medicine Publishing, Tiburon, CA, 1998.

(39)   Donsback, D, Alsleben. M, Systemic Candidiasis and CFS, Don et als, Santa Monica, CA, 1992.

(40)   Donsback, D, Alsleben. M, Systemic Candidiasis and CFS, Don et als, Santa monica, CA, 1992.

(41)   Gilleman, A., Alive Magazine, August, 1998

(42)   Martin, A.W., Healthwatch, Sugar! Be Infromed, R&T. Press, Vol. 1, Issue 10, Pg 1

(43)   Boutros, M., "Pycnogenol®: The Amazing Antioxidant", <u>The Journal of Alternative Medicine,</u> April 1996, 15-26.

(44)   Gabar, B…et al., "Anti-inflammatory and Superoxide Radical Scavenging Activities of a Procyandins containing extract from the bark of pinus pinaster sol and its fractions", <u>Pharma Litt,</u> 1994, 217-220

(45)   Masquelier, J…et al., "Flavonoids et Pycnogenols® "<u>International Journal for Vitamin and Nutrition Research</u> 49 (3): 1979, 307-311.

(46)   Passwater, R, <u>The New Super Antioxidant Plus,</u> Keats Publishing, New Carson, Con, 1992.

(47)   Simon, J "Antioxidants and Their Effects" <u>The American Chiropractor,</u> March/April, 1995, page 22

(48)   Walker, M, "Powerful Antioxidant", <u>Explore,</u> Volume 5, Number 1, 1994, 1-3.

Biography
Dr. A. W. Martin D.C., Ph.D.

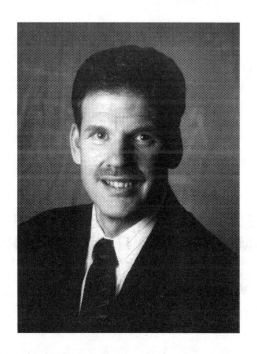

Dr. Anthony W. Martin D.C., Ph.D. graduated from the Canadian Memorial Chiropractic College in 1974. Dr. Martin is a former Vice-President of the Ontario Chiropractic Association and former sports and fitness chairman for the Canadian Chiropractic Association.

Dr. Martin has a Ph.D. in Nutritional Counseling from Lasalle University, Mandeville, Louisiana. For several years he was an associate professor of nutrition at Lasalle

University. Dr. Martin is the author of several books including "**Pycnogenol® - The Bark with the Bite**" and "**The New You - Nature's Way**" and his newest book "**Steps To Fight Chronic Fatigue Syndrome**".

Dr. Martin has been interviewed on several major networks on health related subjects. He is also a personal consultant to several professional athletes including those from the National Football League, Major League Baseball and National Hockey League.

VISIT OUR WEBSITE FOR MORE INFORMATION ABOUT OUR PRODUCTS:

www.martinhealth.com

INDEX

**For credit card orders, please call
1-800-903-3837**

MAIL CHECK OR M.O. + $2.00 SHIPPING PER BOOK
SAFE GOODS,
P.O. BOX 36,
E. CANAAN, CT 06024